Report on Health and Social Subjects No. 46
Nutritional Aspects of Cardiovascular Disease

ISBN 0 11 321875 3

CORRECTION

The national average egg consumption reported in the COMA Report on Nutritional Aspects of Cardiovascular Disease on pages 18 and 74 is incorrect.

Page 18, Table S.2; under column headed "Average household food consumption 1992 (National Food Survey)" and the column headed "Illustrative example of average household food consumption meeting COMA recommendations."

Delete: Eggs   60   1 egg each week

Insert: Eggs   2 (eggs)   2 eggs each week

Page 74, paragraph 2.3.2.10

Delete: "During this period egg consumption halved (falling from about 2.2 eggs/week in 1970 to about 1 egg/week in 1992) . . ."

Insert: "During this period egg consumption halved (falling from 4.7 eggs/person/week in 1970 to 2.1 eggs/person/week in 1992) . . ."

Department of Health
January 1995
LONDON: HMSO

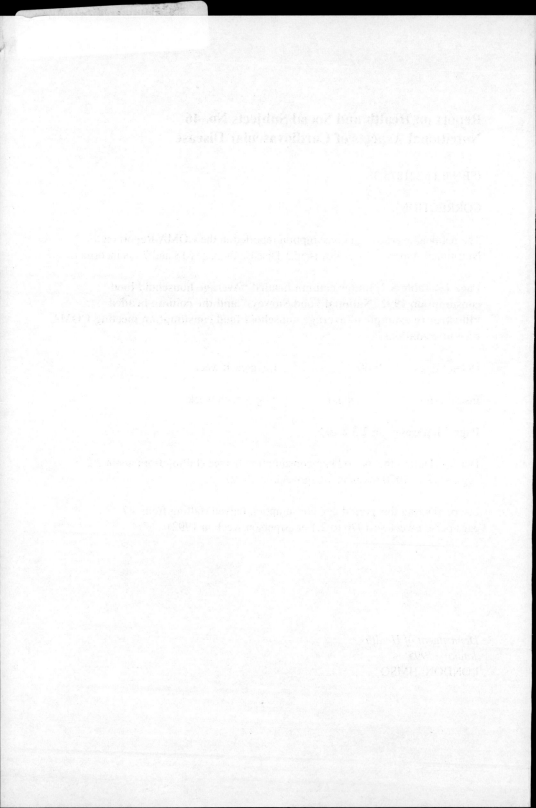

Department of Health

Report on Health and Social Subjects

46

Nutritional Aspects of Cardiovascular Disease

Report of the Cardiovascular Review Group
Committee on Medical Aspects of Food Policy

London: HMSO

Applications for reproduction should be made to HMSO

First published 1994

ISBN 0 11 321875 3

Preface

It is 20 years since COMA first published a report on the relationship between diet and coronary heart disease (CHD). In that time the UK has enjoyed a welcome reduction in deaths due to CHD and to stroke. However the mortality rates in the UK for cardiovascular diseases exceed those of other Western nations which 20 years ago had rates higher than ours, and they remain a major cause of death and of premature death in men and women. Our knowledge of the multiple causes of CHD and stroke remains incomplete, but in the years since COMA's last review of the subject in 1984 there have been substantial advances, helping to refine our understanding of the mechanisms by which diet can influence risk of CHD and stroke. A number of questions remain surrounding the science but finding practical and effective means of changing people's eating habits is the major barrier to implementing what is already known. The recommendation in this Report for research into this aspect is amongst its most important.

The Government's White Paper "The Health of the Nation", published in 1992 contains targets for reductions in CHD and stroke. The dietary and nutritional targets which are included are based on COMA's earlier work. This Report confirms them as appropriate. A novel aspect of this Report is a section specifically on foods, discussing options for dietary change. The Eat Well programme published by the Nutrition Task Force, set up under the 'Health of the Nation', provides a framework for achieving the recommendations of this Report as do the respective strategies in Wales, Scotland and Northern Ireland.

I am grateful to the Chairman and members of the Review Group for the time and effort which they have contributed to making this report.

DR KENNETH CALMAN
Chairman, Committee on Medical Aspects of Food Policy.

iv

Contents

Committee on Medical Aspects of Food Policy Cardiovascular Review Group

Chairman

Professor M G Marmot — Department of Epidemiology and Public Health, UCL Medical School, University College, London.

Members

Professor Dame June K Lloyd — Formerly of Department of Child Health, Institute of Child Health, London.

Dr G J Miller — MRC Epidemiology and Medical Care Unit, The Medical College of St Bartholomew's Hospital, London.

Professor J Shepherd — Department of Pathological Biochemistry, Royal Infirmary, Glasgow.

Professor P Sleight — Cardiac Department, John Radcliffe Hospital, Oxford.

Dr R G Whitehead — MRC Dunn Nutrition Unit, Cambridge.

Professor N Woolf — Department of Histopathology, UCL Medical School, University College London.

Observers

Dr D H Buss — Ministry of Agriculture, Fisheries and Food, London.

Dr P C Clarke — Department of Health, London.

Dr F Harvey (until 1992)	Department of Health, London.
Dr H Kilgore	Department of Health and Social Services (Northern Ireland), Belfast.
Dr R Jacobs	Welsh Office, Cardiff.
Dr V Press (from 1992)	Department of Health, London.
Dr R Skinner	Scottish Office Home and Health Department, Edinburgh.
Mr R W Wenlock	Department of Health, London.

Secretariat

Dr J G Ablett (medical)	Department of Health, London.
Dr M J Wiseman (medical)	Department of Health, London.
Mrs J Caro (administrative) (until October 1992)	Department of Health, London.
Dr S Martin (administrative) (from October 1992)	Department of Health, London.
Miss A Halliday (scientific) (from May 1993).	Department of Health, London.
Mrs E Lohani (technical)	Department of Health, London.

Committee on Medical Aspects of Food Policy

Chairman

Dr K C Calman — Government Chief Medical Officer, Department of Health.

Members

Dr P Aggett — Head of Nutrition, Diet and Health, Institute of Food Research, Norwich.

Professor KGMM Alberti — Professor of Medicine, University of Newcastle upon Tyne.

Dr S Bingham — Non-clinical scientist, MRC Dunn Clinical Nutrition Centre, Cambridge.

Dr J Chambers — Health Education Authority.

Professor F Cockburn — Samson Gemmell Professor of Paediatrics and Child Health, Royal Hospital for Sick Children, Glasgow.

Dr H Denner — Chief Scientist (Food), Ministry of Agriculture, Fisheries and Food, London.

Ms A Foster — Director, Scottish Consumer Council.

Dr G Fowler — Clinical Reader in General Practice, Department of Public Health and Primary Care, Radcliffe Infirmary, Oxford.

Professor J Grimley Evans — Division of Geriatric Medicine, Nuffield Department of Clinical Medicine, University of Oxford.

Dr D Hine — Chief Medical Officer, Welsh Office.

Professor A Jackson	Professor of Human Nutrition, Department of Human Nutrition, University of Southampton.
Professor WPT James	Director, Rowett Research Institute Aberdeen.
Dr M Kemp	Medical Research Council, London.
Dr R E Kendall	Chief Medical Officer, The Scottish Office.
Dr J McKenna	Chief Medical Officer, Department of Health and Social Services, Northern Ireland.
Professor M G Marmot	Professor of Community Medicine, Department of Epidemiology and Public Health, UCL Medical School, University College, London.

Secretariat

Dr M Wiseman (Medical)	Department of Health, London.
Dr S Lader (Medical)	Department of Health, London.
Mr R Wenlock (Scientific)	Department of Health, London.
Mrs M Fry (Administrative)	Department of Health, London.
Dr S Martin (Administrative)	Department of Health, London.
Miss B Ferry (Administrative)	Department of Health, London.

Acknowledgements

The Review Group acknowledge with gratitude the help given by the following in contributing evidence and attending meetings.

Professor C W M Adams (deceased)	Department of Pathology, United Medical and Dental Schools of Guy's and St Thomas' Hospitals, London.
Professor K G M M Alberti*	Department of Medicine, University of Newcastle-upon-Tyne.
Professor D J P Barker*	MRC Environmental Epidemiology Unit, Southampton General Hospital.
Dr D G Beevers*	Department of Medicine, University of Birmingham.
Professor L J Beilin	Department of Medicine, The University of Western Australia, Perth.
Mr K G Berger	Malaysian Palm Oil Promotion Council.
Professor C L Berry*	Department of Morbid Anatomy, London Hospital Medical College.
Dr S Bingham	Dunn Clinical Nutrition Centre, Cambridge.
Professor A Bruce	National Food Administration, Uppsala, Sweden.
Dr E Brunner	Department of Epidemiology and Public Health, UCL Medical School, University College, London.
Dr D A Chamberlain	Cardiology Committee, Royal College of Physicians of London.
Professor F Cockburn*	Department of Child Health, University of Glasgow.

Professor M A Crawford*

Institute of Brain Chemistry and Human Nutrition, Hackney Hospital, London.

Dr G Davey Smith*

Department of Public Health, University of Glasgow.

Professor A T Diplock*

Division of Biochemistry, United Medical and Dental Schools of Guy's and St Thomas' Hospitals, University of London.

Professor J V G A Durnin

Institute of Physiology, University of Glasgow.

Dr P Elliott*

Department of Public Health and Policy, London School of Hygiene and Tropical Medicine, London.

Dr P C Elwood*

MRC Epidemiology Unit (South Wales), Cardiff.

Professor F H Epstein

Institute for Social and Preventative Medicine, University of Zurich.

Dr A B Freeling

Department of Health, London.

Professor J Grimley Evans

Geriatric Medicine Division, University of Oxford.

Professor J S Garrow*

Rank Department of Human Nutrition, St Bartholomew's Medical College, London.

Mr G D Gilbert

The Tropical Growers Association Ltd., London.

Professor S M Grundy

Center for Human Nutrition, University of Texas, Dallas.

Dr S Gupta

Department of Health, London.

Professor M I Gurr*

Maypole Scientific Services, St Mary's, Isles of Scilly.

Dr J Gutteridge*

Department of Anaesthesia and Intensive Care, Royal Brompton National Heart and Chest Hospital, London.

Dr J I Harland

Formerly of The Sugar Bureau, London.

Dr A E Hardman

Department of Physical Education, Sports Science and Recreational Management, Loughborough University.

Dr K W Heaton*

Department of Medicine, University of Bristol.

Professor W P T James

Rowett Research Institute, Aberdeen.

Professor D G Johnston*

Unit of Metabolic Medicine, St Mary's Hospital Medical School, London.

Dr M B Katan

Department of Human Nutrition, Agricultural University, Wageningen, The Netherlands.

Dr A C Keech*

Oxford Cholesterol Study, University of Oxford.

Professor H Keen*

The Metabolic Unit, United Medical and Dental Schools of Guy's and St Thomas' Hospital, London.

Professor Kay-Tee Khaw*

Clinical Gerontology Unit, Addenbrookes Hospital, Cambridge.

Dr M R Law*

Department of Environmental and Preventive Medicine, The Medical College of St Bartholomew's Hospital, London.

Dr J G G Ledingham

Nuffield Department of Clinical Medicine, John Radcliffe Hospital, Oxford.

Ms S Lee

Ministry of Agriculture, Fisheries and Food, London.

Professor A F Lever	MRC Blood Pressure Unit, Western Infirmary, Glasgow.
Ms J Lewis	Ministry of Agriculture, Fisheries and Food, London.
Professor G A MacGregor*	Department of Medicine, St George's Hospital Medical School, London.
Dr A L Macnair*	London.
Professor J I Mann	Department of Nutrition, University of Otago, Dunedin, New Zealand.
Dr H Markowe	Department of Health, London.
Professor T W Meade	MRC Epidemiology and Medical Care Unit, The Medical College of St Bartholomew's Hospital, London.
Professor J R A Mitchell* (deceased)	Department of Medicine, University of Nottingham.
Mr P Morgan	Butter Information Council Ltd., Sevenoaks, Kent.
Professor J N Morris	Department of Public Health and Policy, London School of Hygiene and Tropical Medicine, London.
Dr B Nichols	Van den Berghs and Jurgens Limited, Burgess Hill, West Sussex.
Professor M F Oliver*	Wynn Institute for Metabolic Research, London.
Dr C H Pain	Department of Health, London.
Dr M Rayner	Formerly of The Coronary Prevention Group, London.
Professor G Rose (deceased)	Department of Epidemiology and Population Sciences, London School of Hygiene and Tropical Medicine, London.
Dr J J Segall	London.

Professor P S Sever

Department of Clinical Pharmacology and Therapeutics, St Mary's Hospital, London.

Professor A G Shaper*

Department of Public Health and Primary Care, Royal Free Hospital School of Medicine, London.

Mrs L Stockley

Health Education Authority, London.

Professor J D Swales

Department of Medicine, Leicester Royal Infirmary.

Professor H Tunstall-Pedoe

Cardiovascular Epidemiology Unit, University of Dundee.

Professor N J Wald*

Department of Environmental and Preventive Medicine, The Medical College of St Bartholomew's Hospital, London.

Dr M Waring*

Department of Health, London.

Dr G C M Watt*

Department of Public Health, University of Glasgow.

Professor B Wharton*

Rank Department of Human Nutrition, University of Glasgow.

Mr J Wilkes

Department of Health, London.

Professor C Williams*

Department of Physical Education, Sports Science and Recreational Management, Loughborough University.

* Identifies those who attended discussion meetings with the Panel.

Recommendations

R.1   General

R.1.1   We recommend that people should maintain a desirable body weight (BMI between 20 and 25) as they get older through regular physical activity and eating appropriate amounts of food conforming to the dietary patterns recommended in this Report (S.4).

R.1.2   We recommend that, wherever possible, people should be more physically active. We recommend that schools should offer children a range of physically demanding activities and that those responsible for planning, traffic and environmental policies in town and countryside should consider how they can positively promote walking and cycling (S.5).

R.1.3   We recommend that by the age of 5 years children should be consuming a diet consistent with the recommendations for adults in this Report (S.6).

R.1.4   The recommendations apply to all adults, including most elderly people. We recommend that people should maintain moderate levels of physical activity as they get older, and increase fruit, vegetable and fish consumption. Those whose activity levels are low should do more exercise (S.7).

R.1.5   We do not make different dietary recommendations specifically for smokers, but recommend that people should not smoke (S.1.3).

R.1.6   We recommend that these recommendations are the subject of further review in time (S.1.12).

R.2   Nutrient recommendations

R.2.1   We recommend that the average contribution of saturated fatty acids to dietary energy be reduced to no more than about 10 per cent (S.2.1.2).

R.2.2   We recommend no further increase in average intakes of n-6 PUFA and we recommend that the proportion of the population consuming in excess of about 10% of energy should not increase (S.2.3.1).

R.2.3   We recommend an increase in the population average consumption of long chain n-3 PUFA from about 0.1g/day to about 0.2g/day (1.5 g/week) (S.2.3.2).

R.2.4   We recommend that, on average, trans fatty acids should provide no more than the current average of about 2% of dietary energy and that consideration should be given to ways of decreasing the amount present in the diet (S.2.3.4).

R.2.5   We make no specific recommendations for monounsaturates (S.2.2).

R.2.6   We recommend a reduction in the average contribution of total fat to dietary energy in the population to about 35 per cent (S.2.5).

R.2.7   We recommend that the average dietary intake of cholesterol should not rise (S.2.7).

R.2.8   Complex carbohydrates, and sugars in fruits and vegetables, should restore the energy deficit following a reduction in the dietary intake of fat. We recommend that the proportion of dietary energy derived from carbohydrates should increase to approximately 50 per cent (S.2.8).

R.2.9   We recommend a reduction in the average intake of sodium (principally from common salt (sodium chloride)) by the adult population from the current level of about 150 mmol/day (equivalent to 9g salt/day) to about 100 mmol/day (6g salt/day). We also recommend a similar proportionate reduction in the sodium content of children's diets, but there are currently insufficient data to quantify this (S.2.9.1).

R.2.10 We recommend that food manufacturers, caterers and individuals explore and grasp the opportunities for reducing the sodium content of foods and meals (S.2.9.2).

R.2.11 We recommend an increase in the average intake of potassium by the adult population to about 3.5 g/day (90mmol/day). We also recommend a similar proportionate increase in the potassium content of children's diets, but there are currently insufficient data to quantify this (S.2.10).

R.3   Food recommendations

R.3.1   We recommend that people eat at least two portions of fish, of which one should be oily fish, weekly (S.3.7.3).

R.3.2   We recommend that people use reduced fat spreads and dairy products instead of full fat products (S.3.7.4).

R.3.3   We recommend that people replace fats rich in saturated fatty acids with oils and fats low in saturated fatty acids and rich in monounsaturated fatty acids. An increase in the use of such oils could off-set a reduction in monounsaturates arising from decreased consumption of foods rich in both saturates and in monounsaturates (S.3.7.4).

R.3.4   We recommend that the consumption of vegetables, fruit, potatoes and bread is increased by at least 50% (S.3.7.5).

2

R.4   Research recommendations

R.4.1   We recommend that research is continued and enhanced into the best ways of improving public understanding of, and achieving these recommendations (S.1.9).

R.4.1.1 We recommend that research should be directed towards identifying effective strategies for dietary change, both for populations as a whole and for individuals (1.5.14).

R.4.1.2 More information is needed about the effects of different strategies for achieving dietary change on dietary patterns and on the consequent population risk of disease (1.5.14).

R.4.1.3 We recommend that research is done into the best means of identifying people most susceptible to become obese; into effective strategies to prevent people becoming obese; and into effective treatments for obese people (S.4).

R.4.1.4 Further research is needed on the effect of repeated cycles of weight loss and weight gain on health (5.4.3).

R.4.1.5 Research into the effects of dietary composition on the propensity to obesity should be pursued. More information is needed on the effect of interactions between diet and body fatness on risk (6.8.6).

R.4.1.6 Research into ways and means of decreasing dietary intakes of trans fatty acids is required (S.2.4).

R.4.1.7 Research should be conducted into effective means of implementing the recommendations to reduce population intakes of sodium and increase population intakes of potassium (6.6.10).

R.4.2   We recommend that cardiovascular disease in women and the elderly, and its roots in childhood, should be studied more (S.1.10).

R.4.2.1 Research should be carried out into the definition of optimal growth for children in relation both to their current and to future health; into how nutritional factors contribute to optimal growth and into the nutritional determinants of differences in growth between groups of children in the UK (7.14).

R.4.2.2 More information is needed on the relationship between diet and cardiovascular disease in elderly people, particularly elderly women. More information on the effects of dietary change is required in this age group (8.2).

R.4.2.3 Research is needed to quantify the appropriate intakes of non-starch polysaccharides, sodium, potassium and dietary cholesterol in children (1.5.13).

3

R.4.3   We recommend more research is done into the diverse biological effects of dietary lipids (S.2.5).

R.4.3.1 We recommend that research is continued and enhanced into the different biological effects of different saturated fatty acids, and into practical ways in which such knowledge might improve public health (S.2.1.2).

R.4.3.2 Further research is required on the effects on the serum cholesterol response to particular saturated fatty acids of their position in the triglyceride structure and of LDL receptor activity (6.2.3).

R.4.3.3 The effect of dietary fat and fatty acids on the tendency to thrombosis deserves further research (6.3.2).

R.4.3.4 The effects of n-3 fatty acids on platelet function require further research (6.3.3).

R.4.3.5 The effect of dietary stearic acid on platelet function should be studied (6.3.5).

R.4.3.6 The long term consequences of average intakes by the population of n-6 polyunsaturated fatty acids in excess of about 6% of energy and individual intakes in excess of about 10% of energy should be studied (6.2.5.2).

R.4.3.7 The possibility that dietary cholesterol may influence CHD risk by a mechanism other than through plasma cholesterol requires further investigation (6.2.9).

R.4.3.8 The effects of interactions between dietary cholesterol and fat intakes on cardiovascular risk need further investigation (6.2.9).

R.4.4   We recommend research is carried out to identify the range and effects of various antioxidants in foods and to quantify desirable intakes of dietary antioxidants and/or their food sources (S.2.11).

Summary

S.1   Form of the recommendations

S.1.1   The recommendations in this Report are derived from a wide variety of evidence, which is discussed in detail in the body of the text. This section identifies the key recommendations, and gives a brief summary of their basis.

S.1.2   The main recommendations are given as targets for populations. These are proposed averages for population groups rather than for individual eating. They should not be interpreted as recommended maximum (or minimum) intakes for individuals. The distinction is crucial. To meet a given population dietary target approximately half the population will be expected to consume less than that target, and half more. Some recommendations are more relevant to individuals, and this is made clear in the text.

S.1.3   Except where stated, the recommendations are not applicable to children under the age of 5 years. Separate recommendations are not made for the two sexes. Although the benefit from dietary change, expressed as absolute numbers of heart disease deaths averted, is likely to be greater in men than in women because of the greater incidence of coronary heart disease in men, circulatory diseases are also the major causes of death in women. Furthermore, in the main, these recommendations apply to the overall national diet. Within any country, the same cultural patterns of food consumption can be expected to apply in broad terms to both sexes and to different age groups. These recommendations can be expected to have better than average effects in individuals, who, for whatever reason, are at higher risk of cardiovascular disease. Smokers are at higher risk not only because of their smoking, but also because their characteristic dietary patterns can be expected to lead to increased cardiovascular risk. Smokers might therefore be expected to benefit particularly from following these recommendations. **We do not make different dietary recommendations specifically for smokers, but recommend that people should not smoke.**

S.1.4   Available evidence suggests that for some nutrients, the relation between intake and cardiovascular disease is graded. The lower the intake of saturated fatty acids, for example, the lower the level of plasma cholesterol and the lower the risk of coronary heart disease (CHD). Precise targets might be misunderstood as biologically optimal, but targets are usually a compromise between biological advantage and social, cultural or economic acceptability. We believe that the changes recommended here are moderate and achievable. The combination of recommendations reflects a change to a different, but practicable and enjoyable, dietary pattern. Individually, some recommendations might appear to offer only slight advantage. The cumulative advantage accruing from all our recommendations in an integrated diet offers the prospect of a substantial reduction in risk of cardiovascular disease for the population.

S.1.5   In its 1984 Report, COMA made recommendations not only to Government, but also to the general public, to the food industry and to other sectors of society who might have a role in helping to achieve the recommended changes[1]. This was valuable. We have not followed this procedure because the wider implementation of Government nutrition policy now falls within the remit of the machinery set up under "The Health of the Nation". A key feature of this is the Nutrition Task Force, which has responsibility for drawing up a plan of action to help achieve the specific dietary and nutritional targets in the White Paper, within the context of COMA's wider recommendations. We have understood this role to encompass our present recommendations.

S.1.6   Substantial increases in knowledge have occurred in some areas since 1984. In 1991, some aspects of diet and cardiovascular disease were addressed by the COMA Panel on Dietary Reference Values[2]. We have been able to address in more detail than previously the roles, for example, of sodium, of different saturated fatty acids, and of different classes of polyunsaturates. However our principal recommendations are based on evidence cumulated over decades, much of which was considered by our predecessors and other groups. This evidence is still valid. More recent evidence has provided refinements of understanding of mechanisms, and new insights into practical constraints in achieving change. It is not surprising therefore that the principles behind our conclusions and recommendations are broadly unchanged. Wherever appropriate, new evidence has been incorporated into our recommendations, but it has not warranted a substantive shift in their main thrust.

S.1.7   Our recommendations are given mainly in two forms: as quantitative targets for intake of particular nutrients, and as patterns of food intake. Quantitative targets have public health value in developing and monitoring policy on diet and nutrition. Their precision should not be over-interpreted, as they are based on judgements that balance a number of considerations (see S.1.4). They should therefore be taken together as a cumulative description of qualitative changes in the pattern of nutrient intakes. For most of the recommendations in this Report, the evidence does not suggest a threshold effect above or below which an effect is present or absent. Rather, the relationships between dietary intakes and risk are continuous. The selection of any single figure as a recommendation depends not only on the scientific data, but also on what might practically be achieved within socio-cultural, economic, political and time constraints. The absence of any clear pointers to a single 'optimum' level of intake does not detract either from the strength of the quantitative or qualitative evidence, or from the value of making such recommendations. It should be recognised, however, that these quantified recommendations, though based on the scientific data, are to some extent arbitrary, that is, the result of the exercise of judgement.

S.1.8 Quantitative targets for fat and fatty acids are expressed as proportions of dietary energy. Currently, British adults derive on average about 5% of dietary energy from ethanol in alcoholic drinks. Many individuals, and some population groups, do not drink alcohol at all, and some survey data do not take account of alcohol or of alcoholic drinks. To remove some of the variations, values are sometimes expressed as proportions of food energy (ie excluding ethanol) rather than as total energy. Recommendations for macronutrient intake expressed as a proportion of food energy (ie excluding ethanol) are marginally higher than when expressed as a proportion of total dietary energy. The precision of our recommendations does not warrant such a distinction. These do not therefore take account of the small, variable differences between fat as a proportion of total or of food (ie excluding alcohol) energy. Because the DRV Report met the need for precise reference values, this report has concentrated on the qualitative aspects of change, taking into account the current British diet. Our recommendations, though given as approximate targets, are consistent with the more precise reference values previously published.

S.1.9 Recommendations are also made for changes in the consumption of particular foods and food groups. This has the advantage not only of giving a different set of indices which can help to gauge progress, but also of providing for individuals a semi-quantitative guide of practical value. Advice for individuals is better phrased as patterns of food intake rather than as nutrient targets. Individuals should concentrate on changes in the pattern of intakes of food and foodstuffs. Guidance is given here on the nature and extent of dietary change which would be expected to lead to achievement of the nutrient recommendations. However **we recommend that research is continued and enhanced into the best ways of improving public understanding of, and achieving, the dietary recommendations.**

S.1.10 Fewer data on diet and cardiovascular disease are available for women, children and the elderly than for middle-aged men. It might be argued that extrapolation is not warranted. Such data as are available suggest that the recommendations in this report should apply to the population as a whole. **We recommend that cardiovascular disease in women and the elderly, and its roots in childhood, should be studied more.**

S.1.11 Our recommendations are intended to reduce people's risk of cardiovascular disease. However, many of the nutrients we have considered have effects on health beyond the cardiovascular system. Recommendations which would not be conducive to general, as well as cardiovascular, health would be of limited value. We have not ourselves considered each of these other effects in detail, and have relied on reviews and recommendations from other groups. In general our recommendations are consistent with these other considerations. Our positive recommendations for change (eg reduce saturates) are based on a substantial body of data, with a clear balance in support of the recommendations. Some recommendations are to limit change (eg limit increase in poly-unsaturates). In these cases there may be less rigorous evidence in support of detrimental effects of such changes. However, in the cause of prudence, we have required less evidence for potential harm than for potential benefit when formulating our recommendations. There has been concern that very low levels of plasma cholesterol could lead to increased risk of other diseases. We paid particular attention to the possibility that benefits in reduced incidence of cardiovascular disease, following from dietary recommendations that we and others recommend, could be offset by adverse effects on other diseases. The balance of evidence points clearly to net benefit to health, as well as to decreased cardiovascular disease, from the dietary recommendations in this report.

S.1.12 There are a number of areas of active research on the relation of diet to cardiovascular disease. This research is likely to lead to better understanding of these relationships and their underlying mechanisms. The recommendations here result from the Review Group's judgement, having consulted widely and considered the current evidence. It is our view that if followed, these recommendations would lead to improvement in the health of the nation. The Review Group regard as wholly unrealistic the view that no recommendations can be made until there is absolute certainty. It is unreasonable to expect certainty, which has almost never preceded advances in public health in the past and is unlikely to do so in future. It also seems reasonable to suppose that the national diet will continue to change over the years, as it has in the past, in response to a variety of pressures, of which this Report will be but one. **We recommend that these recommendations are the subject of further review in time.**

S.2 Recommendations for dietary nutrients

This section contains recommendations on nutrients. Section S.3 on Implications for foods is more practical for the lay reader.

S.2.1.1 *Saturated fatty acids* (principally from dairy and meat products and fat spreads) There is strong evidence that increasing or decreasing the contribution of saturated fatty acids to dietary energy is followed by a rise or fall in the concentrations of plasma total and low density lipoprotein (LDL) cholesterol, and in the commensurate risk of coronary heart disease (CHD). The degree of change in cholesterol for a given change in intake of saturates varies between individuals and with the particular fatty acid (see S.2.1.2), but on average is reproducible and can be quantified for groups of people (see 6.2.3). Evidence suggests that the lower the intakes of saturated fatty acids, the lower the risk of CHD. The current average proportion of food energy which is derived from saturated fatty acids is about 16 per cent according to the National Food Survey.

S.2.1.2 There is no evidence that saturates of chain lengths less than 12 or greater than 16 carbon atoms raise plasma cholesterol. Although there is less information, saturates, including stearic acid (C18), appear in addition to have other potentially important effects, such as on platelet activity and the blood clotting system (see 6.2, 6.3). **We recommend that the average contribution of saturated fatty acids to dietary energy be reduced to no more than about 10 per cent. We recommend that research is continued and enhanced into the different biological effects of different saturated fatty acids, and into practical ways in which such knowledge might improve public health.**

S.2.2   *Cis-monounsaturated fatty acids*   Monounsaturates (mainly oleic acid) are a major contributor to total fat intake, and in most foods are the predominant class of fatty acids. These fatty acids currently provide about 15 per cent of food energy according to the National Food Survey (see 2.3). Substitution of saturates by monounsaturates reduces plasma levels of total and LDL cholesterol to about the same extent as substitution by carbohydrates. Substitution by monounsaturates is not accompanied by the fall in HDL cholesterol which occurs with substitution by carbohydrates (see 6.2.4). There is only inconsistent evidence that monounsaturates *per se* actively reduce LDL cholesterol, the observed effects being attributable to concomitant changes in the diet. We did not consider the evidence sufficient to warrant a recommendation specifically to increase monounsaturates because of additional concerns regarding the total amount of fat in the diet but they might usefully substitute for saturates, within an overall total fat ceiling (see S.2.5; S.2.6). **We make no specific recommendations for monounsaturates.**

S.2.3   *Cis-polyunsaturated fatty acids*   The two main classes of cis-polyunsaturated fatty acids (PUFA) – n–3 (principally from oily fish and some seed oils) and n–6 (principally from seed oils and polyunsaturated margarines) – have different biological effects. We have therefore considered them separately. However all polyunsaturated fatty acids have the capacity to undergo oxidation, with potentially adverse effects on the integrity of tissues containing them. This capacity is directly related to the number of double bonds (see 6.5) in the PUFA chain. Many seed oils rich in n–6 PUFA are also naturally rich in vitamin E, a potent antioxidant. Oily fish, a rich source of long chain n–3 PUFA, are not rich in vitamin E. It is prudent for diets containing substantial amounts of PUFA to be adequately supplied with vitamin E. However we have not made a specific recommendation for vitamin E as current evidence is insufficient to quantify the necessary amounts.

S.2.3.1   *n–6 PUFA* (principally from seed oils and polyunsaturated margarines) Apart from their role as essential fatty acids, the n-6 PUFA (mainly linoleic acid) reduce both LDL and HDL cholesterol. There is some evidence that higher intakes of linoleic acid are associated with lower CHD risk (see 6.2.5). On the other hand, there is a largely theoretical concern that linoleic acid-rich diets may increase the tendency to peroxidation of lipids in the artery wall with adverse consequences. Over the last decade there has been a substantial increase in the proportion of food energy which is derived from n–6 PUFA, and the average in the UK is now about 6 per cent. There is not enough observational evidence to provide reassurance of the safety of diets containing more than 9–10% of dietary energy as PUFA over lifetimes. Although n–6 PUFA have tended to substitute for saturates over the last decade, monounsaturates could also substitute (see S.2.6). **We recommend no further increase in average intakes of n–6 PUFA** (see S.2.5). In addition, because there is reason to be cautious about intakes in excess of about 10 per cent of energy, **we recommend that the proportion of the population consuming in excess of about 10% of energy should not increase.**

S.2.3.2 *n–3 PUFA* (principally from oily fish) Long chain n–3 PUFA, ie those with 20 or 22 carbon atoms in their fatty acid chain, for example EPA (eicosapentaenoic acid) and DHA (docosahexaenoic acid), are precursors of the eicosanoids, a family of molecules with a wide variety of important metabolic effects. These fatty acids in the diet can modulate blood platelet activity and the tendency to thrombosis (see 6.3). There is evidence that increasing intake of long chain n–3 PUFA reduces risk of death from recurrent heart attacks, and it is reasonable to suppose a similar effect in relation to first heart attacks. The lowest level of intake required to produce such an effect, or the mechanism involved, is not known but we consider the evidence sufficient to advise a moderate increase. The current contribution of all n-3 PUFA to food energy is less than 1 per cent, with about half from long chain fatty acids. A particularly rich source of the latter is oily fish (eg mackerel, herring, pilchard, sardine, trout, salmon). Consumption of these fish averages 47 g/week and current average intakes of long chain PUFA from oily fish are about 0.1 g/day. About one third of adults consume oily fish in any week, averaging 135 g/week, providing 0.27g/day of long chain PUFA. **We recommend an increase in the population average consumption of long chain n–3 PUFA from about 0.1g/day to about 0.2g/day (1.5 g/week).**

S.2.4 *Trans fatty acids* (mainly from hydrogenated fat in margarines and shortenings and products made from them, eg biscuits, pastries; also from dairy and meat products). A number of recent studies, both experimental and epidemiological, indicate that trans fatty acids, particularly those from margarines and cooking fats, may have undesirable effects not only on plasma LDL and HDL cholesterol, but also on Lp(a) and CHD mortality (see 6.2.5). The average intake of trans fatty acids, at present, is about 2 per cent of food energy, or about 5g per day. **We recommend that, on average, trans fatty acids should provide no more than the current average of about 2% of dietary energy and that consideration should be given to ways of decreasing the amount present in the diet.**

S.2.5 *Total fat* It has been argued that the recommended reduction in saturates could be offset without disadvantage by a similar increase in monounsaturates, thus leaving total fat unchanged. In respect of plasma cholesterol, it seems likely that increasing monounsaturate intake would have no adverse effect. However, there is epidemiological evidence for an association between intake of total fat, as well as of saturates, and CHD mortality. Although the proven association between consumption of saturates and plasma cholesterol can largely account for that association, an additional, independent effect of total fat on CHD risk cannot be ruled out. There are a number of reasons why unrestricted intake of total fat may be undesirable although the evidence for this is not as strong as that for the effect of saturated fatty acids. There is mounting evidence that a higher proportion of energy as fat, irrespective of its composition, predisposes to positive energy balance and hence obesity (see 6.8). There is also some evidence that it may, irrespective of its composition, increase the tendency for blood to clot (see 6.3). Some studies have also found an association between total fat intake and the development of certain cancers, although this remains controversial. In contrast there is no evidence that moderate reduction of fat intakes is associated with ill effects. There are insufficient data to identify an "optimum" level of fat in the diet, though levels less than 10% have been achieved in some circumstances with evidence of benefit[3]. In the UK, a general reduction in total fat intake would also be expected to reduce intake of saturates. We therefore considered it prudent to recommend a specific reduction in total fat consumption. The present average proportion of food energy derived from total fat is about 40 per cent. **We recommend a reduction in the average contribution of total fat to dietary energy in the population to about 35 per cent. We recommend more research is done into the diverse biological effects of dietary lipids.**

S.2.6 *Balance of fatty acids* The recommendations for fatty acids and total fat are interdependent and cannot be considered in isolation of each other. A reduction in the proportion of energy from saturated fatty acids is likely to lead to a concomitant reduction in energy from monounsaturated fatty acids as they are often found in similar foods (see S.3.6). Because of the desirability of reducing the percentage of energy both from saturated fatty acids and from total fat, any increase in the consumption either of monounsaturated fatty acids or of polyunsaturated fatty acids should only be at the expense of the other. The balance of risks and benefits suggests that it would be preferable, given the current composition of the diet, to increase monounsaturates at the expense of polyunsaturates rather than vice versa.

S.2.7 *Dietary cholesterol* (eg from eggs) The influence of dietary cholesterol on plasma cholesterol varies between individuals. The average intake has fallen considerably recently and is now about 245 mg/day (see 2.3.2.10). At this level of intake, an increase in dietary cholesterol can have a significant effect on plasma cholesterol, though quantitatively less than that of saturates. The possibility that dietary cholesterol may influence CHD risk by a mechanism other than through plasma cholesterol requires further investigation (see 6.2.7). **We recommend that the average dietary intake of cholesterol should not rise.**

S.2.8 *Carbohydrates* (eg from bread, potatoes, pasta, rice, sugars) There is no evidence that high intakes of complex carbohydrates – starches and non-starch polysaccharides (NSP) -have adverse effects either generally, or specifically in respect of cardiovascular disease. Although very high intakes of complex carbohydrates are associated with higher plasma concentrations of triglycerides, the clinical significance of this is not clear, and populations consuming such diets have low levels of cardiovascular disease. High intakes of non-milk extrinsic sugars can have undesirable effects on dental health, and in the obese can also predispose to undesirable metabolic effects (see 6.4, 6.8). Restriction of dietary non-milk extrinsic sugars is a sensible contribution to total energy restriction in those who are or are becoming obese. There is evidence that some soluble forms of NSP reduce plasma levels of total and LDL cholesterol. Other forms of NSP, certain starches resistant to digestion in the small intestine, and fruit and vegetable consumption may have other beneficial effects (see S.2.9 and S.2.10). Currently the proportion of energy derived from total carbohydrate is about 45 per cent. **Complex carbohydrates, and sugars in fruits and vegetables, should restore the energy deficit following a reduction in the dietary intake of fat. We recommend that the proportion of dietary energy derived from carbohydrates should increase to approximately 50 per cent.** The COMA Panel on Dietary Reference Values recommended that the population's average intake of non-milk extrinsic sugars should not contribute more than about 10 per cent of energy, and that there should be an increase in the intake of NSP by adults, derived from a variety of foods, from the current average of 12 g/day to 18 g/day.Both these recommendations are consistent with a reduction in cardiovascular risk in the population. We believe it is appropriate for children over the age of 5 years to increase their intake of foods rich in complex carbohydrate, including NSP, so long as their energy requirements are met. While the contributions to energy of starches and sugars recommended above are also appropriate to children over the age of 5 years, there are insufficient data to allow quantified targets for NSP for them.

S.2.9.1 *Sodium* (mainly from common salt)   There is evidence for causal relationships between the consumption of sodium and both the level of blood pressure and the rise in blood pressure with age. The nature of the relationship varies between individuals at least partly in relation to age and prevailing blood pressure, and this may account for the high responsiveness of some individuals which was previously thought to be constitutional "salt sensitivity" (see 6.6). An average reduction of 50 mmol sodium/day (3g salt/day) has been estimated to result in an average reduction in systolic blood pressure of about 3.5 mmHg. A larger effect would be likely to be seen over the longer term as the rise in blood pressure with age was also reduced. Current intakes are about 170 mmol/day in men and 130 mmol/day in women[4]. **We recommend a reduction in the average intake of common salt (sodium chloride) by the adult population from the current level of about 9 g/day (150 mmol/day) to about 6 g/day (100 mmol/day).** Because on average women eat less food than men, this would be expected to represent about 5 g (85 mmol/day) in women and 7 g (115 mmol/day) in men. **We also recommend a similar proportionate reduction in the sodium content of children's diets, but there are currently insufficient data to quantify this.**

S.2.9.2 A reduction (or even an elimination) in the amount of salt added to foods by individuals in cooking or at table would not be sufficient to reach this target and there needs to be a gradual reduction in the amount of sodium, from salt, added to processed foods. **We recommend that food manufacturers, caterers and individuals explore and grasp the opportunities for reducing the sodium content of foods and meals.**

S.2.10 *Potassium*   There is a consistent, but relatively small, body of evidence showing that higher intakes of dietary potassium are associated with lower blood pressures and fewer strokes, in part by mitigating the effect of sodium (see 6.6). The major dietary sources of potassium are potatoes and other vegetables, fruit, meat, milk and other beverages (see 2.3.3.9). Current average intakes are about 3g/day (80 mmol/day) in adults (Gregory *et al*, 1990). **We recommend an** increase in the average intake of potassium by the adult population to about 3.5 g/day (90mmol/day). This would be expected to represent about 3g/day (80 mmol/day) in women and 4g/day (100 mmol/day) in men. **We also recommend a similar proportionate increase in the potassium content of children's diets, but there are currently insufficient data to quantify this.**

S.2.11 *Antioxidant nutrients* A number of essential nutrients, in addition to their actions in preventing classical deficiency diseases, also contribute to the body's defences against oxygen free radicals. Some foods contain other substances which share this property. The principal, but by no means only, nutrients involved are vitamins C and E, and carotenes. Non essential nutrients with antioxidant properties include polyphenolic compounds such as flavonoids. There is increasing evidence from epidemiological and experimental studies that these nutrients may have an important role in modifying susceptibility to atherosclerosis. However, though generally consistent, the body of evidence is still relatively small. Current data are, however, inconsistent in respect of the effective amounts of these nutrients. Epidemiological data suggest that the ordinary diets consumed in parts of Europe are effective but other data suggest that, at least for isolated nutrient preparations, higher doses than can be achieved by diet alone may be necessary. Intervention studies are currently under way or planned which will give important information in this area, particularly concerning the amount of these nutrients which may be required. Pending this information, we have not made quantified recommendations in respect of any specific one of these nutrients. Our recommendations for an increase in starchy foods and fruits and vegetables and substitution of unsaturated vegetable oils for more saturated animal fats would have the effect of increasing the consumption of various antioxidants. We do not recommend supplementation with concentrated or purified preparations as a widespread policy for CHD prevention, as long term safety and efficacy in a variety of population groups has not been demonstrated. In contrast a diet rich in vegetables and fruits is generally regarded as conducive to long term health. **We recommend research is carried out to identify the range and effects of various antioxidants in foods and to quantify desirable intakes of dietary antioxidants and/or their food sources.**

S.2.12 *Alcohol* There is good evidence that alcohol consumption in excess of about 35g/day increases blood pressure and the risk of stroke (see 6.7). There is also evidence that abstainers have a higher risk of CHD than light drinkers (about 10–20g/day). Although this higher risk is partly due to abstainers including individuals who have given up alcohol for reasons of ill health, this does not account for the whole effect. There is evidence for a direct effect of ethanol increasing HDL cholesterol, and some alcoholic beverages also contain other active principles, in particular phenolic flavonoids in red wine (see 6.5). The sensible drinking levels (approximating to 24g ethanol daily for men and 16g daily for women) do not take account of the protection afforded from CHD, but they are consistent with this. Habitual drinking in excess of this increases the risk of raised blood pressure, and of stroke, and of other serious health and social problems. We do not recommend consumption of alcohol as a policy for CHD prevention because of the risk of adverse effects.

S.3   Implications for foods

S.3.1   The nutrient content of the average diet in Britain differs in a number of respects from that recommended in this report (Table 2.1). Therefore, for the recommendations to be achieved in the context of a nutritionally adequate diet, there would have to be major changes to the national average pattern of food consumption in Britain so that the diet contains significantly less saturated and total fat and sodium, and significantly more fruits and vegetables, complex carbohydrates, non-starch polysaccharides (NSP – fibre) and potassium. There are as many different ways of responding to the recommendations as there are individual diets. It seems likely however that any changes in the national pattern of consumption would result from a variety of changes across the whole range of foodstuffs rather than drastic changes in one or two. On this assumption the population as a whole would consume less fatty meat and meat products, high fat dairy products and full fat spreads etc. In addition, lower fat and lower salt versions of more foods would need to be developed and little salt added to food 'at the table.' A substantial increase would take place in the average amount of potatoes, bread, pasta and other carbohydrate rich foods eaten, in order to replace the energy that would be lost if fat intake was reduced.

S.3.2   The changes that individuals might make to their own diet depends on their current dietary pattern, which varies widely across the population, and on a number of other circumstances. Many individuals within the population have already made changes to their diets over the past decade, and this is reflected in the increased consumption of skimmed and semi-skimmed milks, low fat spreads, lower fat meat products and other reduced fat alternatives (see 2.3.2). However, although this has resulted in a fall in the average percentage of energy from saturates, there has been no change in the average percentage of energy from fat.

S.3.3   The aim of this report is to recommend changes to the average diet of the population, not specific dietary changes for individuals. Nevertheless some guidance for individuals may be helpful. A healthier diet may consist of changes not only in the proportional amounts of different foods, but also in the type of foods consumed. In practice, it is likely that individuals who wish to change will use various combinations of these approaches. Table S.1 shows some examples of how the fat and saturated fatty acid content of the diet can be reduced by substituting one food or meal with a lower fat alternative. For instance, eating a reduced fat Cheddar type cheese sandwich with low fat spread in place of a "normal" Cheddar cheese sandwich with butter could "save" 19g fat and 15g saturates.

S.3.4   Data from MAFF's National Food Survey (NFS) give a good picture of the current average diet of the British population that is eaten at home. Table S.2 shows the amounts and types of food currently consumed and gives an example of how they might change consistent with the nutrient recommendations in this report. The table is not a prescriptive diet of foods for individuals, but is one example of how future NFS results might look if all COMA's recommendations were met. Adjustments to consumption outside the home cannot be illustrated in

Table S.1:   The fat and saturated fatty acid saving from a variety of dietary substitutions

• The recommendations in this Report imply a reduction in national per capita average consumption for total fat of around 15g per day, and for saturated fatty acids of around 11g per day.

Food swap	Fat saving g/portion	Saturated fatty acid saving g/portion
1 bowl breakfast cereal with whole milk exchanged for 1 bowl breakfast cereal with semi-skimmed milk	2	1
1 bowl breakfast cereal with whole milk exchanged for 1 bowl breakfast cereal with skimmed milk	4	2
1 egg fried in oil exchanged for 1 egg boiled	3	1
2 rashers grilled bacon and 1 fried egg exchanged for 1 bowl breakfast cereal with semi-skimmed milk and 2 slices toast with low fat spread	28	11
2 slices bread with butter exchanged for 2 slices bread with low fat spread	11	9
2 slices bread with butter exchanged for 2 slices bread with polyunsaturated margarine	0	8
Cheddar cheese sandwich with butter exchanged for reduced fat cheddar type cheese sandwich with low fat spread	19	15
Cheddar cheese sandwich with butter exchanged for cheddar cheese sandwich without butter	18	11
1 thick and creamy fruit yoghurt exchanged for low fat fruit yoghurt	3	1
2 digestive biscuits exchanged for 1 banana	7	3
1 chocolate bar exchanged for 1 apple	15	9
1 packet crisps exchanged for low fat crisps	5	1
2 grilled sausages exchanged for 2 low fat grilled sausages	13	5
1 pork chop, lean and fat grilled exchanged for 1 pork chop, lean only	19	7
100% beefburger in a bun exchanged for low fat beefburger in bun	5	2
Cheeseburger (100% beef) in bun exchanged for 100% beefburger in bun	5	3
White fish in batter, fried in oil exchanged for white fish, steamed or baked (no added fat)	33	3
Baked potato with butter exchanged for baked potato with low fat spread	8	8
Baked potato with butter exchanged for baked potato with baked beans	15	10
Baked potato with cheddar cheese exchanged for baked potato with cottage cheese	16	10
1 medium portion chips fried in oil exchanged for 1 medium portion boiled potatoes	12	1
Sponge cake with butter icing exchanged for currant bun with low fat spread	11	3
Pie with 2 crusts exchanged for pie with 1 crust	6	2
Egg mayonnaise exchanged for egg with reduced fat mayonnaise	31	4
4 mugs tea/coffee with whole milk exchanged for 4 mugs tea/coffee with semi-skimmed milk	2	1

the same way, due to the present lack of information on this part of the diet. On average food and drink bought and consumed away from home account for roughly 10% of energy intake. The balance between foods may differ significantly from home consumption, but some at least of the changes shown in Table S.2 might also be expected to be reflected in habits when eating out.

S.3.5   As well as the example presented in Table S.2, many other strategies for reducing intake of saturated and total fat from the diet could be envisaged. For example, the recommendations could be met by removing from the diet most dairy products or most meat, or many of the fattier convenience products (e.g. cakes & biscuits, meat products, potato products etc.), or most fat spreads and oils, while changing the rest of the diet to a comparatively small degree. Replacing fatty meat and meat products with fish, low fat dairy products, or beans and pulses would be possible options. However these strategies would lead to extreme changes in the consumption of other foods – for example, a very large increase in the consumption of bread and potatoes – in order to meet energy needs. None of these approaches would be likely as average diets for the whole of the population, but they do indicate that groups or individuals within the population can choose different approaches in moving towards the nutritional recommendations. The example shown in Table S.2 is based on a number of less extreme changes across a wider range of food groups in the diet.

S.3.6   The report recommends a substantial reduction in the average amount of sodium, principally from common salt, consumed each day (by about 3g salt per day). On average, adults add around 1.5g salt (600mg sodium) to the foods they consume each day. Reducing or eliminating the practice of adding salt during cooking or at the plate would go a substantial way towards meeting the salt recommendation. But for the recommendation to be met there would also be a significant reduction either in the consumption of foods which make a significant contribution to salt intake, such as bread, meat products, processed cereal products and processed vegetables, or in the amounts of salt used in their manufacture. Simply reducing the consumption of these foods to the levels consistent with the salt recommendations without any change in their composition would be unrealistic, requiring a substantial compensatory increase in the quantities of (unsalted) potatoes, rice or pasta. The example in Table S.2 therefore assumes some reformulation of bread, meat products, processed vegetables and breakfast cereals to produce a 30% reduction in the amount of salt added to them. The changes in food consumption illustrated in Table S.2, together with the suggested reformulations, could lead to a further reduction of salt intake of 1.2g (470 mg sodium), on average, each day. But in the long term, salt levels of these products might be reduced further (a 50% reduction would reduce salt intakes by 1.8g (720mg) each day compared with current intake), or perhaps more likely, a wider selection of foods, such as soups, sauces etc, with a reduced sodium content might be developed. Manufacturers are already producing many processed foods with lower levels of sodium, and these can be used to help reduce the total amount of salt in the diet. A key issue will be balancing salt reduction against palatability and safe keeping qualities. Table S.3 shows some changes that individuals could make to their own diets to help reduce their salt intake.

S.3.7 In Table S.2 the number of portions given is a national average. For any individual food, some people eat more and some less: in general men, active people and adults more; children, sedentary and elderly people and women less. Individual preferences also matter: the exact changes that individuals might make to their diets will depend on the foods they like and the amounts they are already eating. Some foods may not be eaten at all by a substantial number of people. The main changes in national average consumption illustrated in the example in Table S.2 are described below.

S.3.7.1 *Milk and dairy products*   In the example, the total amount of milk is little changed but a further switch to semi-skimmed or skimmed milk is shown. Young children under the age of two should be given whole milk rather than semi skimmed or skimmed milks as a main drink. A change of this type could reduce average fat intake by just over 2g/day and saturates by about 1.5g/day. The example also includes a reduction in the amount of cheese, on average by 50%, to produce a fat saving of 2.5g/day and a saturates saving of 1.5g/day. This also helps reduce salt intake. A change in the types of cheese consumed for lower fat varieties, (e.g. a change to reduced fat Cheddar type cheese, cottage cheese, or Edam type cheeses), would mean that total cheese consumption might be greater than in the example.

S.3.7.2 *Meat and meat products*   The example shows no change in the amount of carcase meat consumed, but a switch towards lean meat. For those individuals who eat fatty meat, trimming visible fat could reduce total fat intake by about 3g/day, and saturates by just under 2g/day. The main change suggested for this food group is an average reduction by around 50% in the amount of meat products and dishes consumed. This might mean eating 3 fewer portions of meat products each week, or eating smaller portions of meat products (e.g. thin sausages instead of thick; thinner spread of paté on bread etc.), or mean incorporating less meat (and more vegetables, pulses or potatoes) into manufactured meat dishes. If a move to lower fat varieties were assumed, the total quantity consumed would not reduce as much. In practice, a combination to suit individual needs and preferences is likely. The change shown for meat products and dishes might lead to a reduction of around 5.5g fat/day and just over 2g saturated fat/day. At the same time it would reduce the amount of salt consumed, since many are currently fairly high in salt. The example in Table S.2 also assumes some reformulation of these products to contain around 30% less salt than they currently do.

S.3.7.3 *Fish*   An increase in the amount of oily fish (such as mackerel, herring, sardine, trout, salmon, pilchard) in the diet to around one portion per week is shown. This would increase intake of long chain n-3 PUFA. Consumption of other fish and fish products is assumed not to change. **We recommend that people eat at least two portions of fish, of which one should be oily, weekly.**

S.3.7.4 *Fat spreads and oils*   The example shows a switch from margarines and butter to low and reduced fat spreads without any reduction in the amount of fat spread used. There has already been a major increase in the number of indi-

Table S.2: Illustrative example of changes to National Food Survey results if COMA's recommendations were met. The figures represent national averages, not recommendations for individuals (see Section S.3). Food and drinks provided and eaten away from home would be additional to the amounts shown below.

Food Group	Average household food consumption 1992 (National Food Survey)		Illustrative example of average household food consumption meeting COMA recommendations		Comment
	g/person/week*	Rough equivalent in terms of portions	g/person/week*	Rough equivalent in terms of portions	
Milk	1960 (ml)	1 glass whole milk plus 1 glass semi skimmed milk each day	2140 (ml)	½ glass whole milk and 1¼ glasses semi skimmed milk each day	Continues trend to low-fat milk. Cheese consumption is currently steady.
Other milk and cream	260 (ml)	1 tablespoon cream each day	130 (ml)	½ tablespoon each day	
Cheese	115	filling for 2-3 sandwiches each week	60	filling for 1-2 sandwiches each week	
Carcase beef and lamb	210	2 portions each week	210	2 portions *lean* meat each week (trimmed of visible fat)	For carcase meat the amount is left unchanged but a switch to leaner meat assumed; for meat products the example shows reduced consumption with no change in fat content.
Pork and poultry	300	3 portions each week	300	3 portions each week	
Other meat and meat products	440	7 portions each week	220	3½ portions each week (assumes 30% reduction in sodium content)	
Fish and fish products	140	1 portion white fish or fish products plus ½ portion oily fish	190	1 portion white fish or fish products plus 1 portion oily fish	In effect this means doubling the number of people eating sardines, salmon, etc in any week
Eggs	60	1 egg each week	60	1 egg each week	Assumes no change
Butter	40	spread for 3 slices bread each day	20	spread for 1½ slices bread each day	
Margarine	80	spread for 1 slice bread each day	40		
Low and reduced fat spreads	50	spread for 1 slice bread each day	120	spread for 2½ slices bread each day	Continues switch to low-fat spreads and move from butter/margarine/lard to vegetable oils for cooking
Vegetable oils	50	4½ tablespoons each week	100	9 tablespoons each week	
Other fats	25	1½ tablespoons each week	10	¾ tablespoon each week	

Table S.2 (cont): The figures represent national averages, not recommendations for individuals (see Section S.3).

Food Group	Average household food consumption 1992 (National Food Survey)		Illustrative example of average household food consumption meeting COMA recommendations		Comment
	g/person/ week*	Rough equivalent in terms of portions	g/person/ week*	Rough equivalent in terms of portions	
Potatoes	900	1 small portion potatoes (2 egg sized potatoes) each day	1260	1 medium portion potatoes (3 egg sized potatoes) each day	Assumes 50% increase in main categories; present trends are for fruit to increase (mainly juice) but potatoes and bread falling
Potato products	170	each week either: 2 potato croquettes or 1 medium portion chips	80	each week either: 1 potato croquette or small portion chips	
Vegetables and products	1130	2–3 portions each day	1690	4 portions each day (assumes 30% reduction in sodium content of processed vegetables)	
Fruit and products	930	1½ pieces fruit each day	1290	2 pieces fruit each day	
Bread	750	3 slices each day (of which 1½ slice wholemeal)	1130	4½ slices each day of which 1 slice wholemeal (assumes 30% reduction in sodium content)	
Buns, cakes and biscuits	290	3–4 biscuits each day	145	1–2 biscuits each day	Assumes 50% reduction, with no change from current composition
Breakfast cereals	130	1 bowl each day	130	1 bowl each day	Assumes no change
Other cereals	285	1 serving pasta or rice each day	285	1 serving pasta or rice each day	
Sugar and preserves	200	6 teaspoons sugar each day or (or good spread for 2 slices bread)	190	5 teaspoons sugar each day or (or thin spread for 2 slices bread)	Continues trends on sugar/ preserves and move to low-calorie soft drinks. Assumes small reduction in consumption of confectionery.
Soft drinks (containing sugar)	720 (ml)	2 cans each week	360 (ml)	1 can each week plus any amount sugar free drinks	
Chocolate confectionery	35	1 small bar each week	30	¾ small bar each week	Consumption of soft drinks and confectionery is probably heavily understated because much is bought for consumption away from home.
Sugar confectionery	15	3 boiled sweets each week	15	3 boiled sweets each week	
All other foods	440	2 tablespoons pickle or dressing each day	440	2 tablespoons pickle or dressing each day	Assumes no change

*Unless otherwise stated

Table S.3   The sodium and salt saving from a variety of dietary substitutions.

The recommendation in this Report is for a reduction in national average sodium intake of around 1g (roughly 2.5g salt) for adults, and less for children.

Food swap	Sodium saving g/portion	Salt saving g/portion
1 portion old potatoes boiled in salted water with 1 portion old potatoes boiled in unsalted water	0.1	0.3
1 portion peas boiled in salted water with 1 portion peas boiled in unsalted water	0.1	0.2
1 portion canned peas with 1 portion peas boiled in unsalted water	0.2	0.4
1 portion carrots boiled in salted water with 1 portion carrots boiled in unsalted water	0.05	0.1
1 portion spaghetti boiled in salted water with 1 portion spaghetti boiled in unsalted water	0.4	1.0
1 portion rice boiled in salted water with 1 portion rice boiled in unsalted water	0.4	0.9
1 portion regular baked beans with 1 portion low-salt baked beans	0.3	0.8
1 portion salted peanuts with 1 portion fresh peanuts	0.2	0.5
1 packet regular potato crisps with 1 packet potato crisps with no added salt	0.3	0.7
Saving when salt is not added to food at home	0.6	1.5

viduals using lower fat spreads over the past few years, and this trend is likely to continue. The change shown in the example could save around 3g fat and 2g saturates each day. For those who choose to change entirely to low fat spreads, the savings will be correspondingly larger. It would theoretically be possible to meet the recommendations with a reduction (or even an elimination) of fat spreads from the diet but this is unrealistic given that the example assumes increased bread consumption. An increase in the amount of vegetable oils consumed is also compatible with the recommendations. The example assumes that this increase is of a vegetable oil rich in monounsaturated fatty acids (eg rapeseed oil, olive oil) to avoid any further increase in polyunsaturated fatty acids. The recommendations do not call for a change in monounsaturates. However because monounsaturated fatty acids tend to be found in similar foods to saturated fatty acids, consumption of monosaturates would fall with a reduction in consumption of foods rich in saturates. Increased availability and use of spreads and oils rich in monounsaturated fatty acids would help to offset this. **We recommend that people use reduced fat spreads and dairy products instead of full fat products. We recommend that people replace fats rich in saturated fatty acids with fats and oils low in saturates and rich in monounsaturates.**

S.3.7.5 *Potatoes, vegetables, fruit and bread*   The example includes an approximate 50% increase in the levels of vegetables, fruit, potatoes and bread compared with current intakes. This is equivalent to a total intake of approximately 6 portions of vegetables or fruit, 2 portions of potatoes or pasta or rice and 4 slices of bread each day, which would replace the energy lost in the diet from the reduction in other foods. These levels of intake result in an increase of carbohydrate to around 50% of energy as recommended and would also lead to increased intakes of antioxidants. **We recommend that the consumption of vegetables, fruit, potatoes and bread is increased by at least 50%.**

S.3.7.6 The example in Table S.2 also assumes reformulation of bread and processed vegetables to reduce salt content by 30%. In other examples that were devised, where salt content was left unchanged, the amount of bread was much less, with the shortfall in energy being replaced by potatoes, pasta or rice instead.

S.3.7.7 A 50% increase in consumption of these foods would also lead to an increase in the levels of NSP, potassium and some antioxidant nutrients in the diet. The example in Table S.2 results in an increase in NSP to around 15g/day. This would probably be consistent with adults eating the Dietary Reference Value for NSP of 18g/day, and children eating less.

S.3.7.8 *Cakes and biscuits*   The example shows a 50% reduction in the average consumption of these foods. This is equivalent to eating two fewer biscuits each day. This might reduce fat intake by about 3.5g/day and saturates intake by about 1.5g/day, and would also reduce intake of non-milk extrinsic sugars. Manufacturers have developed alternative versions with less fat or sugar. Successful marketing and further development of these alternatives might offer the opportunity of helping to meet the recommendations without so large a change in total consumption.

S.3.7.9 *Sugars, preserves and confectionery* Table S.2 shows reductions of about 5% in the amount of sugar and preserves, and 20% in chocolate confectionery, in line with previous recommendations for the reduction of non-milk extrinsic sugars. Continuation of the current trends to substitute sugar-free varieties for conventional soft drinks with sugar would also help to achieve this recommendation.

S.3.8   Overall, the changes to the national diet illustrated above would meet the population nutrient recommendations set out in this report. Table S.4 shows the effect on other nutrients in the diet. Energy intakes would be essentially unchanged while intakes of most vitamins and minerals are increased or maintained. There is a small reduction in retinol equivalents but this is not nutritionally significant. Intakes of trans fatty acids are likely to remain around current levels.

S.3.9   At the prices recorded in the 1992 National Food Survey the changes illustrated in Table S.2. would not have raised the cost of the average diet. Indeed there would be a slight decrease from £14.39 to £14.10, although the 2% difference is not significant. Obviously some people would pay more and some less than the average prices used.

S.4   Recommendations for the prevention of obesity

Excessive accumulation of body fat inevitably follows chronic energy consumption in excess of expenditure, and is associated with higher mortality from CHD and stroke, as well as higher morbidity from a number of conditions. This association, independent of smoking and mediated partly through higher levels of blood pressure and plasma cholesterol, is particularly important at higher levels of fatness (see 5.4). Obesity, defined conventionally as a body mass index above 30, is increasing in the UK. In 1991 16% of adult women and 13% of adult men in England were obese. The proportion increases with age up to age 64: 25% of women and 19% of men aged 55–64 were obese. No single dietary constituent uniquely causes the energy imbalance leading to obesity. However a diet relatively rich in fat appears to be particularly conducive to so called "passive caloric overconsumption" due to its poor satiating properties and high energy density (see 6.8). Lower levels of physical activity also contribute to positive energy balance. Treatment of established obesity is difficult, and prevention is therefore especially important. **We recommend that people should maintain a desirable body weight (BMI between 20 and 25) as they get older though regular physical activity and eating appropriate amounts of food conforming to the dietary patterns recommended in this Report. We recommend that research is done into the best means of identifying people most susceptible to become obese; into effective strategies to prevent people becoming obese; and into effective treatments for obese people.**

Table S.4:   The nutrient composition of different diets

Nutrient	Current national average diet (a) Average intake/ person/day	Example shown in Table S.2 Average intake/ person/day
Energy (kcal)	1960	1906
Total fat (% energy)	40	35
Saturates (% energy)	16	11
Monounsaturates (% energy)	15	14
Polyunsaturates (% energy)	7	7
Carbohydrate (% energy)	46	50
NMES[1] (% energy)	13	11
NSP[2] (g)	12	15
Retinol equivalents (µg)	1150	1010
ß-carotene (µg)	1750	2450
Thiamin (mg)	1.26	1.50
Riboflavin (mg)	1.64	1.63
Niacin (mg)	25.6	26.5
Folate (µg)	249	293
Vitamin B_6 (mg)	1.8	1.9
Vitamin B_{12} (µg)	5.0	4.9
Vitamin C (mg)	54.0	65.7
Vitamin D (µg)	2.97	3.66
Vitamin E (mg)	8.2	9.5
Calcium (mg)	840	863
Iron (mg)	10.3	11.2
Magnesium (mg)	232	252
Copper (mg)	1.1	1.2
Zinc (mg)	7.9	8.0
Phosphorus (mg)	1130	1140
Potassium (mg)	2540	2860
Sodium (mg)	2530	2070

(a) Taken from National Food Survey 1992

[1] Non milk extrinsic sugars   [2] Non-starch polysaccharides (fibre)

S.5   Recommendations for physical activity

S.5.1   The level of physical activity is an important modifiable determinant of risk of obesity. In addition, a low level of physical activity is independently associated with increased risk of CHD. Increasing activity reduces CHD risk. The Task Force on Physical Activity, established under the Health of the Nation is examining the possibilities of setting specific targets for levels of physical activity. Meanwhile, **we recommend that, wherever possible, people should be more physically active.** Activity need not be sporting, but some exercise should be quite vigorous, although regulated according to individual capacity. Everyday activities such as walking, cycling and using the stairs if performed regularly can be beneficial, and can be modified to suit different levels of ability. Such simple activities should be a regular part of daily life.

S.5.2   Adults who have been sedentary should increase their activity levels gently and progress steadily, and respond promptly to any ill effects. The hazards of increased physical activity are outweighed by the benefits.

S.5.3   A life-long commitment to exercise is more likely to develop in those who have established the habit in childhood. **We recommend that schools should offer children a range of physically demanding activities and that those responsible for planning, traffic and environmental policies in town and countryside should consider how they can positively promote walking and cycling.**

S.6   Recommendations for children

Many processes linked with the development of cardiovascular disease have their origins in childhood. Growth of the fetus and infant may also be implicated in the development of cardiovascular and other diseases in adult life. The dietary and other recommendations for adults do not apply to children below the age of 2 years, for whom adequate energy intake for growth remains paramount. Between the ages of 2 and 5 years a flexible approach to the timing and extent of dietary change should be taken. **We recommend that by the age of 5 years children should be consuming a diet consistent with the recommendations for adults in this report.**

S.7   Recommendations for older people

The recommendations apply to all adults including most elderly people. However, the special needs and small appetites of some elderly people increase the chance of energy and nutrient deficiencies if inappropriately stringent diets are advised. **We recommend that people should maintain moderate levels of physical activity as they get older, and increase fruit, vegetable and fish consumption.** Those whose activity levels are low should do more exercise. These are of particular importance, and have considerable benefits, not just for prevention of cardiovascular disease, but also for other major chronic diseases and for quality of life. Since the absolute risk of disease is high in this age group the potential for benefit is also high.

1. Introduction

1.1   Background

On two previous occasions the Committee on Medical Aspects of Food Policy (COMA) has reported on diet and cardiovascular disease[1,18]. Among the recommendations of the 1984 report was one for a continuing review of the evidence. This report is a product of that review.

1.2   Terms of reference

"To review the 1984 COMA Recommendations on Diet and Cardiovascular Disease, and to advise COMA on any change considered necessary in the light of new knowledge."

1.3   Meetings and way of working

1.3.1   The Review Group met thirteen times and conducted its review in two parts. The first part involved assessing expert opinion on the current status of the 1984 report. Experts in the UK and elsewhere were sent a copy of the 1984 report, and asked to comment on its conclusions and recommendations in the light of recent advances. This led to the second part of the review and a series of discussion meetings with invited experts. The topics considered at these meetings were identified in the previous trawl and comprised: lipids; sodium, potassium and blood pressure; natural history of atherosclerosis; free radicals and antioxidant nutrients; non-cardiovascular and all causes mortality in relation to prevention of cardiovascular disease; recommendations for elderly people; carbohydrates; obesity; physical activity; soft water. Following these discussion meetings, the Review Group met 4 times to consider and complete this Report. The Review Group are grateful to the many individuals involved at both stages of the trawl and discussions, all of whose names are included in the list of contributors on pages 6–9.

1.4   Cardiovascular disease

1.4.1   *Coronary Heart Disease (CHD)* may manifest itself clinically in a number of different forms, including:
- stable angina
- unstable angina
- acute myocardial infarction ("heart attack")
- sudden death – with or without a history of previous infarction and/or preceding chest pain

1.4.2 *Stroke* is the sudden localised loss of brain function due either to failure of the blood supply (ischaemia) or haemorrhage, and lasting longer than 24 hours. Severe generalized cerebral damage occurring as a result of oxygen lack should not be regarded as stroke. In the UK, approximately 85 per cent of cases of stroke are due to ischaemia, of which the major cause is thrombosis in the arteries supplying the brain; the remainder are due to emboli (clots which have travelled from the heart or other blood vessels). Haemorrhagic stroke results from rupture of the arterial wall due to wall disease or aneurysm.

1.4.3 *Peripheral vascular disease* Peripheral vascular disease is almost entirely manifest as disease of the aorta, and of the iliac and leg arteries. With the exception of a particular kind of smoking related arterial disease (Buergher's disease), reduced blood supply is rarely a problem in the arms. Peripheral vascular disease often coexists with CHD. The main clinical manifestations are pain in leg muscles on effort (intermittent claudication), and rest pain, which may require amputation, when arterial insufficiency is more severe.

1.4.4 *Burden of disease* Cardiovascular diseases (CHD and stroke) are the major causes of death in men and women. In 1990, CHD accounted for 30% of male deaths, and 23% of female deaths. Stroke accounted for 15% of female deaths and 9% of male deaths. Coronary heart disease and stroke are also important causes of premature (i.e. before age 65) mortality; in men, CHD caused 37% of deaths in the 55–64 age group in 1990. Eight percent of all male deaths and 2% of all female deaths are due to premature death from CHD (see 2.1).

1.5 **Perspectives**

1.5.2 *Fundamental principles* This report focuses on the **nutritional** contribution to mortality and morbidity from cardiovascular disease and to their prevention. It is based on several propositions:

- In principle premature mortality and morbidity from the major cardiovascular diseases are preventable, at least in part.

- Diet is a major and modifiable cause of cardiovascular disease. Diet can therefore be considered central to prevention, but the cause of vascular disease is multifactorial; therefore a preventive strategy must include action on other causes, in addition to diet.

- Cardiovascular diseases are the major causes of death, and are major causes of morbidity, in the population of the United Kingdom and other industrialised countries. These diseases and their risk factors are so widespread in the population that recommendations for their prevention should be aimed at the whole population.

- The dietary changes recommended here to the general public are also likely to have a favourable impact on other diseases.

1.5.3 *CHD and stroke risk can be reduced* Three types of evidence suggest that CHD and stroke are preventable.

(i)   There are large international differences in incidence and mortality rates which are not fixed. When peoples migrate from one country to another, their rates of CHD and stroke change towards that of their new country[5-9].

(ii)   There have been rapid changes over time in rates of mortality from, and presumably in the rates of occurrence of, CHD and stroke. In the USA CHD mortality rates have declined by more than 40 per cent over the last 15–20 years, suggesting an environmental/lifestyle rather than a genetic cause for the decline (see 2.1.5.2).

(iii) A great deal of knowledge has accumulated on the causes of these diseases with impressive evidence that many causes can be avoided; and that even though causes may act over decades, their effects may be partially reversible in a few years.

1.5.4   *Prevention and reduction of risk*   Were it possible to place individuals into two groups, one of which would definitely succumb to cardiovascular disease (i.e. at 100% risk) and the other which would definitely not (i.e. zero risk), prevention could then be appropriately targeted only at those at risk.

1.5.5   Such a clear distinction is not possible. Currently, the likelihood of developing cardiovascular disease can only be categorised in retrospect as zero or 100 per cent. Future risk can only be estimated as lying somewhere between those two extremes, and all individuals will appear to be at some level of risk, though some will be higher than others. However, with present knowledge of risk factors (see below), it is possible to predict risk of subsequent disease to a substantial degree. The chance of sustaining disease increases as the level and number of risk factors increases, but it is never a certainty. Better understanding of constitutional factors, including genetic, which predispose individuals to develop cardiovascular diseases would be a valuable aid to targeting preventive measures.

1.5.6   The aim of prevention is **to reduce the probability** of subsequent disease. Just as it is not yet possible to predict precisely who will and who will not develop the disease, it is not possible to guarantee its avoidance in every individual who takes preventive action – though the population as a whole will benefit.

1.5.7   An example of the inevitable consequences of this imprecision of prediction is the observation that some individuals with a strong family history of CHD can smoke, take no exercise, eat a high fat diet and still not develop cardiovascular disease. In retrospect, action to change lifestyle would therefore not have benefited these people, at least in respect of cardiovascular disease. Some people who adopt a healthy lifestyle nevertheless suffer from cardio-vascular disease. Both these are exceptions to a general pattern. As reviewed in this Report, the evidence is strong that diet and other risk factors do affect risk of disease. The proportionate change in risk is more or less independent of its initial level and specific nature.

1.5.8   Recommendations which successfully lower morbidity and mortality from cardiovascular disease but result in increased rates from some other diseases, and therefore to no reduction in overall mortality, might not be helpful. The aims of prevention are to increase quality of life at all ages, and to reduce age specific, and especially premature, mortality. The Review Group therefore paid special attention to the possibility that there might be adverse consequences of dietary change to prevent cardiovascular disease.

1.5.9   *Strategy of prevention*   Prevention should be part of good medical practice. Usually this seeks to identify people at particularly high risk of CHD or stroke and modify their risk by lifestyle changes or drug treatment ("high risk approach"). It is the classical approach of preventive medicine, and deals with individual high risk patients. The "population approach" seeks not only to reduce the occurrence of high risk states but also to modify existing average population levels of risk. These two strategies are complementary. The European Atherosclerosis Society[10] recommends intervention for individuals with a plasma cholesterol higher than 6.5 mmol/l, currently 23 per cent of British adults. If our recommendation to reduce dietary saturated fatty acids to about 10 per cent of dietary energy were implemented, mean plasma cholesterol levels would decline by about one eighth and the proportion requiring individual intervention according to EAS criteria would decline from 23 per cent to 6 per cent.

1.5.10   As a means of improving public health, the population approach has the potential for delivering greater gains across the whole population. Two examples are given based on blood pressure and serum cholesterol (Figures 1.1 and 1.2). Figure 1.1 is based on data from the 350,000 white males screened for possible entry into the US Multiple Risk Factor Intervention Trial (MRFIT) (Marmot and Shipley, unpublished). The excess deaths are calculated on the assumption that the CHD death rate of men with a systolic blood pressure less than 110 is the basal rate. The higher death rates at higher levels of blood pressure can be "attributed" to blood pressure. A "high risk" approach that sought to detect and treat those with systolic blood pressure greater than or equal to 170 mm Hg would potentially save only a small proportion of these excess deaths. Although CHD risk rises with blood pressure, most deaths attributable to a raised blood pressure occur in that part of the population, the majority, with only moderately higher pressures. The risk is graded even within this "normal" group. Only an approach that lowers blood pressure of most of the population could reduce the majority of the deaths attributable to blood pressure. The same principle applies for serum cholesterol (Figure 1.2). This emphasises the importance of a strategy aimed at the whole population.

1.5.11   A strategy aimed at the whole population has an important feature in common with one aimed at finding and treating high risk people. If successful they both reduce the risk of the **current** generation of adults. In addition, however, a population strategy has the potential to reduce the risk of **subsequent** generations.

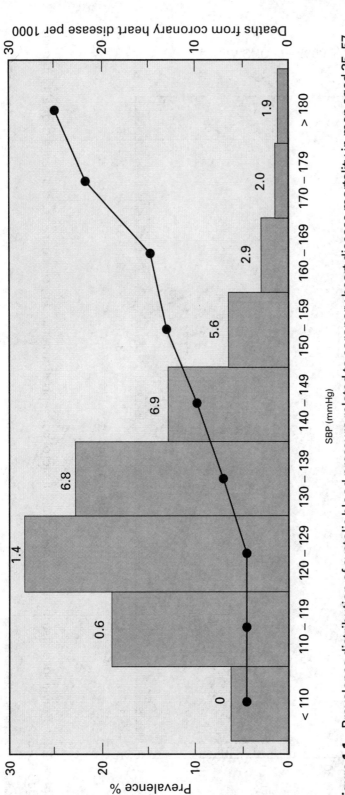

Figure 1.1 Prevalence distribution of systolic blood pressure related to coronary heart disease mortality in men aged 35–57.

Baseline systolic BP and 6-year age-adjusted CHD mortality in 347,923 men aged 35-57 free of MI at baseline (MRFIT)

Number above each bar represents the attributable deaths per 10,000 population over 6 years.

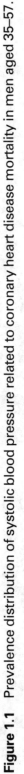 Deaths from CHD per 1000 (●——●)

Source: Marmot and Shipley (unpublished)

29

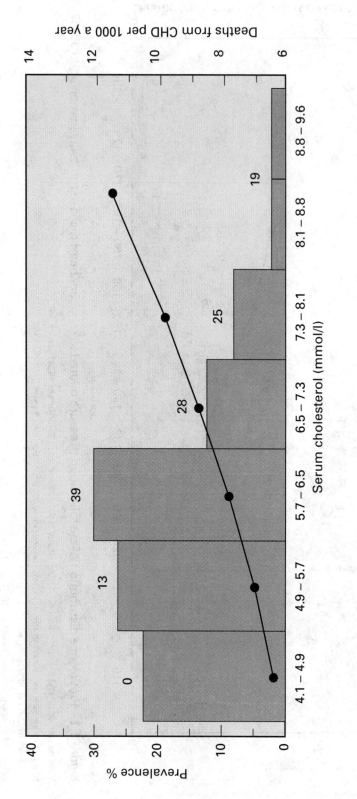

Figure 1.2   Prevalence distribution of serum cholesterol concentration related to coronary heart disease mortality in men aged 55–64.

Deaths from CHD per 1000 per year (●———●)

Number above each bar represents estimate of attributable deaths per 10,000 population per 10 years.

Source: Calculated from Rose[11]

1.5.12 Evidence linking plasma cholesterol to cardiovascular disease comes from epidemiological, clinical and laboratory studies. Clinical trials have mainly been confined to studies of middle aged men, while epidemiological studies have been concerned with comparisons among various populations including migrants, and longer term prospective studies within populations. The trial data have been contrasted with the data from epidemiological studies[12-14]. While both sets of information address the broad issue of plasma cholesterol and cardio-vascular disease, principally CHD, there are important differences between them. Atherosclerosis is a process which takes decades to develop. Middle aged men are likely already to have developed significant coronary atherosclerosis, even though they may have no symptoms. Interventions in these people (to reduce existing high plasma cholesterol) are therefore likely to have less effect on the development and outcome of atherosclerosis than lifelong alterations in diet (to prevent high plasma cholesterol occurring). Nevertheless meta-analysis of trial data indicates that much of the benefit in respect of CHD mortality predicted from epidemiological studies is achieved by about five years[12,13]. It is difficult to imagine experimental methods to explore the lifelong effect on true primary prevention of atherosclerosis (as opposed to prevention of symptoms or death in people with atherosclerosis) beyond those already employed in the wide variety of epidemiological studies. These data are strong, consistent and show the characteristics of a causal relationship between plasma cholesterol and CHD mortality[12,13]. Trial data provide important information, but such data address a limited aspect of CHD and do not negate conclusions drawn from the extensive epidemiological evidence.

1.5.13 Fewer data on diet and cardiovascular disease are available for women and the elderly than for middle-aged men. Although premenopausal women have a lower CHD risk than men, after the menopause the difference in risks narrows. It might be argued that extrapolation is not warranted. Such data as are available suggest that the recommendations in this report should apply to the population as a whole. In general we believe that failure to extrapolate for example from men to women or from middle aged to older people results in more rather than less harm. This failure has in the past led to the undertreatment of such groups until adequate data eventually emerged, for example failure to offer thrombolysis to women or to elderly people, or aspirin to women with transient cerebral ischaemia. Therefore, where data are inadequate and in the absence of evidence that some harm might result we have preferred to use the same guide-lines as for other subgroups. We recommend that cardiovascular disease in women and the elderly should be studied more in the future. In addition there is sometimes insufficient information on current or desirable intakes for instance of non-starch polysaccharides (NSP), sodium, potassium, and dietary choles-terol, for children. We recommend that research is done into quantifying appro-priate intakes of these nutrients in children.

1.5.14 In addition, some studies have addressed the efficacy of studies designed to change dietary behaviour[14]. In contrast to the strong evidence for the effects of diet on plasma cholesterol and of reduction of plasma cholesterol on CHD risk, these studies show that the actual change in plasma cholesterol following prescription of a particular diet is smaller than expected. This strongly suggests that the actual diet was not the same as that prescribed over the period of the study. We recommend that research should be directed towards identifying effective strategies for dietary change, both for populations as a whole and for individuals. In addition, more information is needed about the effects of different strategies for achieving dietary change on dietary patterns and on the consequent population risk of disease.

1.5.15 *Secondary prevention and treatment* Lifestyle modification is also likely to be beneficial in people who already have symptomatic disease. Although the recommendations in this report apply to those with symptomatic disease, their medical management is not part of this report.

1.5.16 There have been proposals for routine plasma cholesterol screening of the population in order to find people at high risk because of their level of plasma cholesterol. As indicated above, cardiovascular risk is not determined solely by the level of plasma cholesterol, and although valuable for a small proportion of the population, such an individual approach is expensive, wasteful of resources and unlikely to have a large population benefit unless accompanied by a whole population approach to prevention. In addition, because individuals may be at high risk for reasons unrelated to plasma cholesterol, a low level of plasma cholesterol might erroneously imply low overall risk, and so paradoxically have a detrimental effect by false reassurance. For example a diabetic patient with a "normal" cholesterol might well have a greater risk of CHD than a non diabetic with a raised cholesterol. Yet lowering cholesterol in the diabetic is associated with a reduced risk of CHD. The cost effectiveness of plasma cholesterol testing was examined by the Standing Medical Advisory Committee, who published a consultation document in 1990[15]. As a result, the Department of Health advises that cholesterol testing should only be undertaken as part of a comprehensive CHD prevention programme, taking into account the presence of other risk factors[16].

1.5.17 *Causes, risk factors, and variations of occurrence* The term risk factor is used in various ways[17]. Risk factors for cardiovascular disease can be divided into:

- inherent biological traits such as age, sex and family history that cannot themselves be altered;

- modifiable physiological characteristics that affect the likelihood of future occurrence of disease (eg blood pressure, plasma cholesterol or fibrinogen, obesity, diabetes);

- behaviours (eg diet, smoking, lack of physical activity, alcohol consumption) that may be associated with cardiovascular disease because of their links with characteristics such as blood pressure or plasma cholesterol, or via other mechanisms;

- social characteristics such as social class or ethnic group that mark out differences in rates of occurrence of disease without identifying mechanisms, whether due to differences in behaviour, to other social and cultural factors, or to genetic or other constitutional factors;

- other environmental influences that may be primarily physical or psychological. For example, cold weather, unemployment, bereavement and severe emotional stress may contribute to risk.

Genetic factors can modify the impact of behavioral factors such as smoking or diet, or act independently on physiological function as in familial hyperlipidaemia.

1.5.18 *Multiple risk factors* Risk can be expressed as proportionate or absolute difference in disease associated with difference in risk factors. The multiple risk factors for cardiovascular disease make independent contributions to relative risk. The proportionate decrease in CHD for a given decrease in plasma cholesterol level appears to be independent of the level of other risk factors. Smoking appears to double the risk of CHD whatever the level of plasma cholesterol. However because people with a high plasma cholesterol have a greater absolute risk than people with a low cholesterol level, the doubling of risk due to smoking will have a greater absolute effect in people with high plasma cholesterol. To be fully effective, therefore, a strategy must deal with multiple risks.

1.5.19 Although a number of factors are known to influence risk of cardiovascular disease, they are still insufficient to explain all the variation in cardiovascular risk between people. Unknown factors must also operate. Many factors, both known and unknown, are likely to have contributed to the decline in CHD death rates since the early 1970s. There are no good data on past trends in plasma cholesterol or blood pressure in the UK, but the National Food Survey provides data on dietary trends. While intake of saturates has declined, and that of polyunsaturates has increased, total fat as a percentage of energy has been more or less constant. Over the last decade the prevalence of obesity has increased dramatically and that of smoking has declined. It is the net effect of these known – and unknown – risk factors which impinge on CHD rates. The decline in CHD deaths in the USA and Australia has been greater than in the UK and their CHD rates are now substantially lower than in the UK. It is therefore reasonable to aim for a faster rate of decline than currently seen in the UK. Prevailing CHD death rates are lower in countries such as France, with broadly similar known risk factors, suggesting that at least some unknown risk factors are of considerable importance.

1.5.20 It is possible to calculate the reduction in cardiovascular deaths which would be predicted to follow a reduction in plasma cholesterol in the population (see 5.2.3). In addition, there have been a number of efforts to estimate the effect of a reduction in plasma cholesterol on life expectancy. Some have attempted to take account of changes in multiple risk factors. Estimates vary widely and there is no consensus on which, if any, of the different models is best. Most of these attempts have not taken into account possible reductions in non-fatal as well as fatal coronary heart disease and hence do not provide an estimate of disease-free life expectancy. We are, therefore, not able to give a precise quantitative estimate of the effect on healthy life expectancy of the changes recommended here.

1.5.21 Dietary factors play a central role in the causation or prevention of cardiovascular disease, although they are by no means the only factors of importance. In order to reduce effectively and efficiently the community burden and individual suffering from cardiovascular diseases, action needs to be directed at other important risk factors. The concentration on diet in this Report should not, therefore, be taken to imply that factors primarily outside the specific remit of this Group (eg smoking) are not also of fundamental importance. In this Report we have touched on those factors which inter-relate substantially with diet while other important but less related factors may have received less attention or been omitted. Our recommendations are intended to complement those which address important social, regional and ethnic variations in cardiovascular disease, which require a different public health focus.

1.6   Form of the report

1.6.1   This Report is COMA's third review of the relationship between diet and cardiovascular disease. The first, in 1974, made qualitative dietary recommendations, while the second suggested quantitative targets[1,18]. Since those Reports were published another COMA Panel has proposed dietary references values for fat and carbohydrate, as average population figures[2]. The Government has adopted the dietary reference values for saturated fatty acids and total fat as targets to help achieve a reduction in deaths from coronary heart disease and stroke as part of a strategy for health, in the White Paper "The Health of the Nation"[19].

1.6.2   Numerical targets are valuable. Targets provide an objective means of assessing progress. However when there is no objective evidence of a clear biological threshold for an effect, the selection of the quantified target, as opposed to qualitative advice, must involve judgement. This arbitrary nature of some targets does not detract from their validity or value. The association between plasma cholesterol and rate of occurrence of coronary heart disease (CHD), for example, is graded and continuous. Evidence from a large number of studies in industrialised countries shows that the lower the plasma cholesterol level the lower the risk of disease. Evidence from China shows that the continuous nature of the relationship extends to lower levels of plasma cholesterol than are commonly seen in Britain[20]. A similar conclusion is likely to apply to saturated fatty acids: within the range studied, the lower the intake the lower the risk of heart disease.

1.6.3   Public health recommendations should take into account not only what may be biologically optimal, but also social, cultural or economic acceptability. Differences in numerical targets among different expert groups may reflect their judgement of the practical constraints as much as their view of the biological relationships. The scientific evidence has to be balanced against the changes in national diets that may be practicable and achievable. Targets which equate to the very much lower fat and saturates intakes, such as in Japan or China, would be less easily achieved and not necessarily desirable in Europe. **We give numerical targets recognising that they are what may be feasible currently within the UK and not necessarily what may lead to the lowest attainable rate of cardiovascular and other diseases.** Our targets are sometimes approximate rather than precise to reflect the graded nature of some relationships, and the arbitrary nature of the selected target.

1.6.4   The main targets are presented as desirable means for the population. These are not what every individual should eat. The distinction is crucial. A target of an **average** 35% of food energy from fat in the diet is not an indication that no individual should exceed that level. If as now, the standard deviation of the proportion of dietary fat is of the order of 5%, then for only 2.5% of the population (2 standard deviations above the mean) to exceed 35% of food energy from fat, the population average would have to be 25%. A population target is most likely to be achieved if the distribution of dietary intake of the whole population shifts, rather than simply if alterations are confined to subgroups of the population. Unfortunately it is not yet possible to identify with sufficient certainty those who will benefit most – or least – from such a strategy. Such information, when forthcoming, may render different strategies more practicable. All individuals, and particularly those at high risk – for whatever reasons – are likely to benefit from changes in line with these recommendations.

1.6.5   It is reasonable for government and others concerned with healthy patterns of eating for the whole population to think in terms of numerical targets for nutrients. It is less reasonable for individuals to plan their behaviour according to such numerical targets. It is not feasible for individuals, however expert in nutritional science, to know with any certainty where they lie on the population distributions of intakes and requirements of the various relevant foods or nutrients. We therefore also present our recommendations in the form of patterns of eating for the general public.

1.6.6   The many factors which contribute to the development of cardiovascular diseases reflect a variety of mechanisms underlying the pathology. Not every aspect of these mechanisms is directly affected by diet. However, diet may have an impact on pathogenesis at a number of stages in the pathological process in a variety of ways. It is only possible to view the effects of diet when set in a broad context. The Group decided to review the underlying processes – for instance in biochemistry and pathology – from a wider standpoint than the purely nutritional, and to describe them in comprehensive, though not exhaustive, detail.

1.6.7   As with any judgements based on scientific evidence, these conclusions on policy represent best judgement based on current evidence. There is nothing immutable about the evidence, which is incomplete and sometimes inconclusive. Nevertheless, many of the recommendations in this Report are similar to those in previous Reports from COMA. During the review of evidence, some submissions sent to us questioned previous COMA recommendations in the light of more recent evidence. We have thoroughly reviewed the evidence which led to those recommendations, and new evidence which has accumulated since they were published. Where there are similarities, these are a positive reinforcement of those recommendations. We have addressed in the text the specific areas of new information, which in general complement rather than contradict previous knowledge. In some cases, evidence was considered insufficient to form the basis of new recommendations, though it has sometimes been possible to give qualitative advice. The reasons behind apparent differences from previous recommendations or their rationales which might be of particular interest are given below.

1.6.7.1 *Sodium*   In 1984 COMA recommended that intake of common salt should not be increased further and consideration should be given to ways and means of decreasing it. In 1991 the COMA Panel on Dietary Reference Values was unable to estimate the average requirement for sodium in the UK[2]. Their considerations, which focused on requirements for sodium as an essential nutrient, did not directly address "*optimum*" intakes in respect of the link between dietary sodium and blood pressure. Rather the Reference Nutrient Intake for sodium reflects the lowest average levels of intake in the UK population compatible with nutritional adequacy, within socio cultural constraints[2]. There has been a substantial new body of evidence since 1984 relating dietary sodium to blood pressure, and the debate since 1991 has helped to clarify apparent inconsistencies (see 6.6). This Report has specifically addressed the role of sodium in modulating blood pressure in the population, and our recommendation for a reduction is consistent with, though less stringent than, the Reference Nutrient Intake. It is likely that, were the population's average sodium intake to fall to the Reference Nutrient Intake, the benefit in terms of reduction of blood pressure and so of stroke and CHD would be greater, and the risk of inadequate intake of sodium remain virtually non-existent. However, we believe the likelihood of such a reduction being achievable in the UK population within the next decade to be small.

1.6.7.2 *Dietary cholesterol*   In 1984, COMA made no specific recommendations on the consumption of dietary cholesterol. Over recent years, dietary cholesterol intake has fallen considerably (see 2.3). In 1991, the COMA Panel on Dietary Reference Values, while noting the effects of dietary cholesterol on plasma cholesterol, did not identify a specific parameter by which to define a reference value and consequently, did not set one. We have addressed the dietary intake of cholesterol in the specific context of cardiovascular disease, and in particular of plasma cholesterol, with a view to making recommendations (see 6.2). Our conclusions are the same as those of the Panel on Dietary Reference Values. We recognize that the contribution which dietary cholesterol makes to plasma cholesterol is less than that of dietary saturates. Our recommendation that dietary cholesterol should not rise is consistent with these conclusions, and follows from our specific remit.

1.6.7.3 *Total fat*   The recommendation in this Report for total fat is essentially identical to that in COMA's Report on Dietary Reference Values. In the latter, the recommendation on total fat is an inescapable consequence of the recommendations to reduce saturates, and not to increase intakes of any other class of fatty acids[2]. This rationale remains valid. Furthermore there is a well described association between total fat intake and CHD mortality (see 6.1). Much of this association can be attributed to co-correlation with dietary saturates and an effect of total fat intake on CHD independently of its composition has not been demonstrated. However the combined evidence for mechanisms whereby total fat might contribute, independently of its composition, to such an association make it unwise to exclude such a possibility. In addition, there are a number of strands of evidence which argue for benefit from restriction of total fat, irrespective of its composition. Some of these data, eg on total fat and the clotting pathway (see 6.3) or on the possible link between dietary fat and the development of some cancers, were available during previous considerations, but individually provided insufficient grounds for a specific recommendation on total fat. In contrast there has been a substantial increase in data in other areas. In particular, evidence that diets rich in fat are particularly prone to encourage positive energy balance and so the development of obesity has accumulated (see 6.8). Together these data argue for a specific benefit from restraint in dietary fat intake. The current recommendation for total fat therefore rests not only the evidence available previously, but also on more recent data.

2. The Current Position

2.1 Cardiovascular disease

2.1.1 *Cardiovascular disease mortality* In 1990 Coronary Heart Disease (CHD) accounted for 27% of all deaths in the United Kingdom and stroke for 12%. Between 1986 and 1990 CHD accounted for 24% of all years of life lost up to age 75 in males in England and Wales, and stroke for 4%. The corresponding figures for females were 12% for CHD and 6% for stroke. In 1990 83% of deaths occurring from CHD in the UK were in people over age 65 and the corresponding figure for stroke was 92%. CHD accounts for 30% of all male deaths in the UK compared with 23% of all female deaths, whereas stroke accounts for 15% of all female deaths and 9% of male deaths (see Figure 2.1).

Figure 2.1 Distribution of deaths by sex and selected cause. United Kingdom 1990

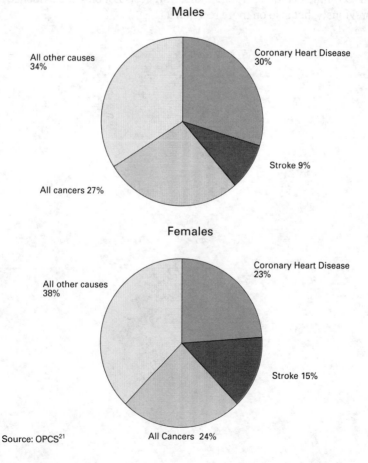

Males

Coronary Heart Disease 30%

Stroke 9%

All cancers 27%

All other causes 34%

Females

Coronary Heart Disease 23%

Stroke 15%

All Cancers 24%

All other causes 38%

Source: OPCS[21]

2.1.2 Figure 2.2 shows the difference in relative importance of the major causes of death between age-groups. In males the relative importance of CHD increases with age up to the group aged 55–64 years, in whom it causes 37% of deaths, after which it decreases, causing 29% of deaths in those aged 75–84 years. In females CHD becomes increasingly important with age. Cancer is more important in younger women but declines in importance in comparison with cardiovascular disease with increasing age. The relative importance of stroke increases with increasing age in both males and females.

Figure 2.2 Distribution of deaths by age group by sex and selected disease, United Kingdom 1990

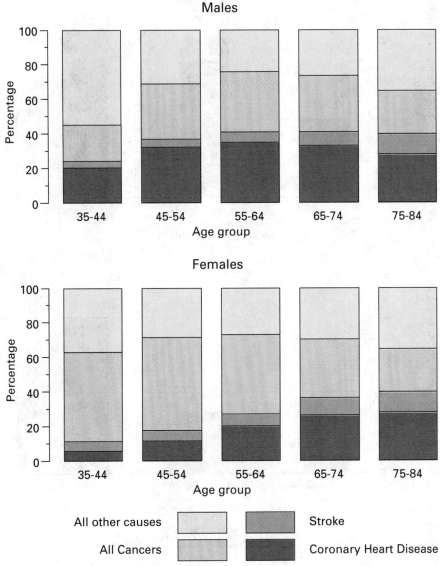

Source: OPCS[21]

2.1.3 *Cardiovascular disease morbidity* The rates for patients consulting GPs in England and Wales for CHD and Stroke are shown in Figure 2.3 (note the use of different scales for the two diseases). These give some indication of the morbidity caused by these diseases though they are only an indirect measure. Patient consulting rates are generally higher, and the increase in consulting rate with age is less marked for CHD than for stroke. The consulting rate is higher in all age-groups for both diseases for males.

Figure 2.3 Patients consulting GPs by sex and age. England and Wales 1981/82

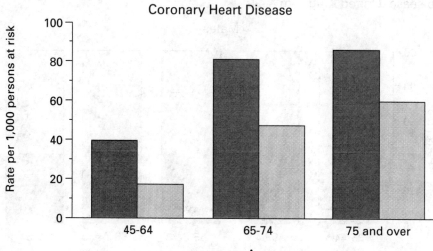
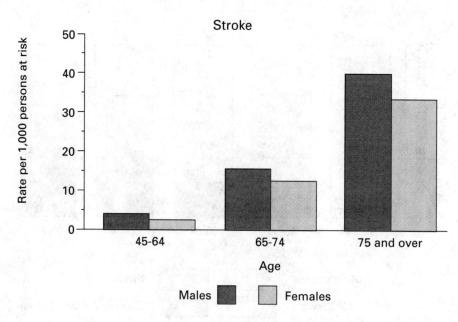

2.1.4   Figure 2.4 shows the differences in hospital episodes for patients being treated for CHD and Stroke. The rates for these age-groups are higher for men than for women for both diseases. For stroke the episode rate increases sharply with age, while for CHD the rate for males at age 85 and over is below that at 75–84 and there is little increase in the episode rate for females between these age-groups.

Figure 2.4 Ordinary and day case episodes by sex and age, England 1989/90

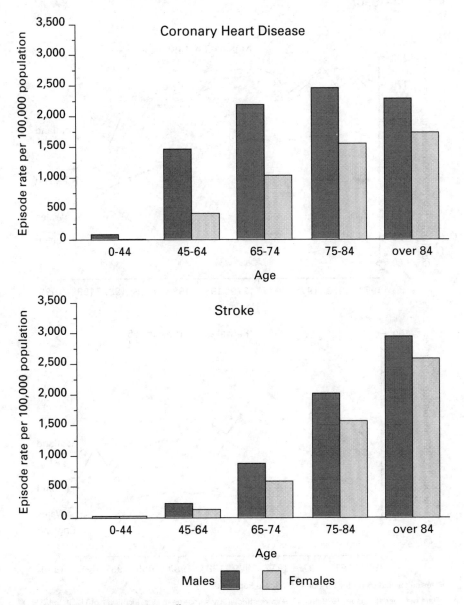

Source: DH Hospital Episode Statistics[23]

2.1.5   *Secular trends*

2.1.5.1 Figures 2.5a to 2.5d show the secular trends in the four countries of the UK between 1972 and 1989. Three year rolling averages have been calculated based on data from 1971 to 1990. Longer term trends and more detailed analysis for those aged 35–64 are given in Appendix B. Figures 2.5a to 2.5d show death rates for females remaining below those for males throughout the period 1972–1989. For CHD, death rates changed little over the period to 1978 with

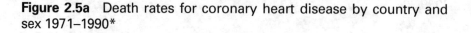

Figure 2.5a Death rates for coronary heart disease by country and sex 1971–1990*

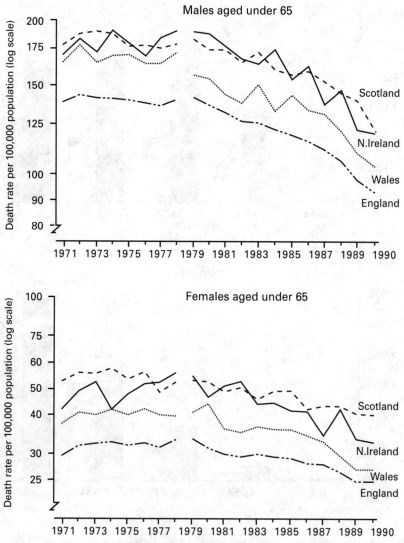

Rates calculated using the European Standard Population

*Data between the years 1978 and 1979 were affected by a change in classification from ICD8 to ICD9

Source: OPCS[21]; Registrar General's Offices of Scotland and N. Ireland

subsequent fall, particularly marked for males aged under 65. For stroke (Figures 2.5c and 2.5d), rates fell over the whole period, with a faster decline in the under 65 groups than for all ages. The rates for the different countries of the UK have followed broadly similar patterns. Death rates for Scotland and N. Ireland have remained consistently higher than those in England and Wales.

Figure 2.5b Death rates for coronary heart disease by country and sex 1971–1990*

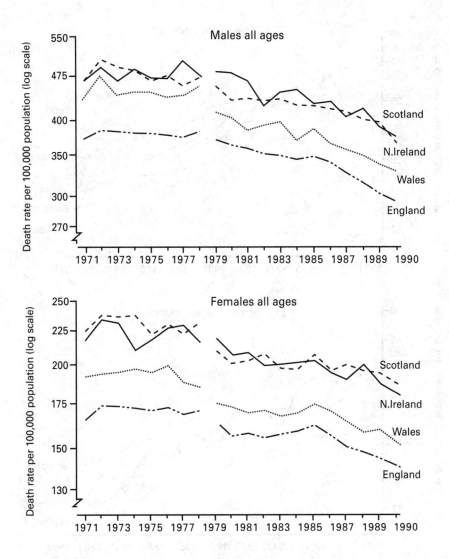

Rates calculated using the European Standard Population

*Data between the years 1978 and 1979 were affected by a change in classification from ICD8 to ICD9

Source: OPCS[21]; Registrar General's Offices of Scotland and N. Ireland

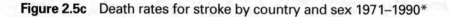

Figure 2.5c Death rates for stroke by country and sex 1971–1990*

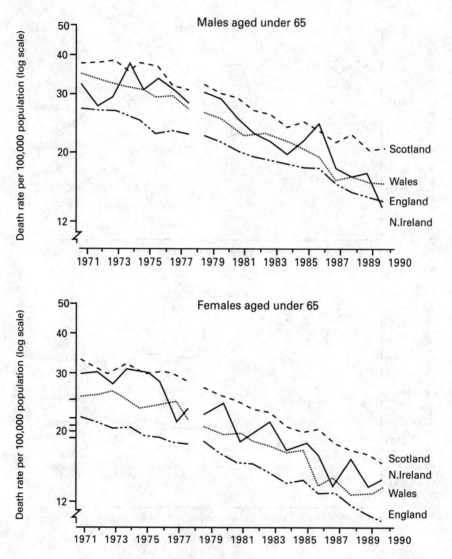

Rates calculated using the European Standard Population

*Data between the years 1978 and 1979 were affected by a change in classification from ICD8 to ICD9

Source: OPCS[21]; Registrar General's Offices of Scotland and N. Ireland

Figure 2.5d   Death rates for stroke by country and sex 1971–1990*

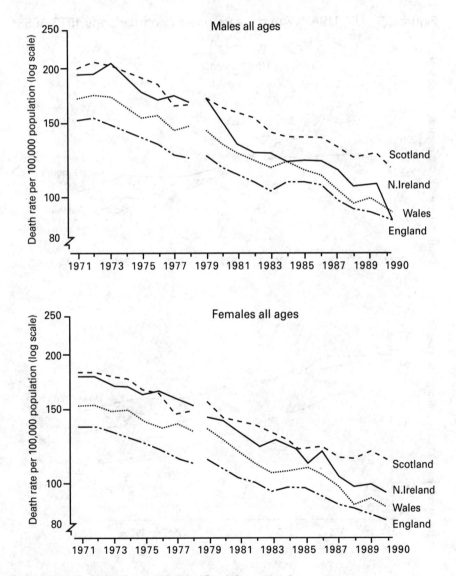

Rates calculated using the European Standard Population

*Data between the years 1978 and 1979 were affected by a change in classification from ICD8 to ICD9

Source: OPCS[21]; Registrar General's Offices of Scotland and N. Ireland

2.1.5.2 *The UK compared to the USA and Australia*   Figure 2.6 shows trends in CHD and stroke standardised mortality rates for the USA, Australia and the UK. The decline in CHD mortality in the UK began later than in the USA and Australia, and although the UK rate was initially lower, these two countries now have considerably lower rates than in the UK. The comparisons are less striking for stroke but, nevertheless, reductions in stroke rates for the UK have not been as rapid as in either the US or Australia. Australia, while starting with a higher mortality rate in 1970, had achieved a rate considerably lower than the UK by 1988.

Figure 2.6   UK, USA & Australian mortality comparisons 1970–1988*

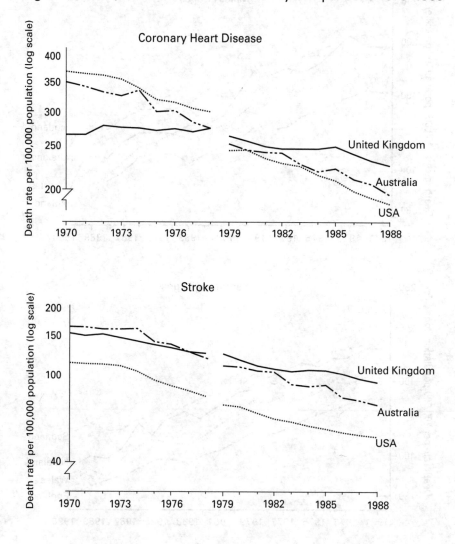

All person rate calculated using the European Standard Population

*Data between the years 1978 and 1979 were affected by a change in classification from ICD8 to ICD9

Source: WHO[24]

2.1.5.3 *Trends in death rates from all causes*   Figure 2.7 shows death rates from all causes in the period 1979–1988 in the UK, USA and Australia. Declines in all causes mortality have been substantial in all countries, and have occurred at the time of reduction in several major risk factors for cardiovascular disease. Declines in intake of saturated fatty acids, and in smoking have been reported in all 3 countries.

Figure 2.7 Standardised death rates*: UK, USA & Australia All persons, All Causes 1970–1988

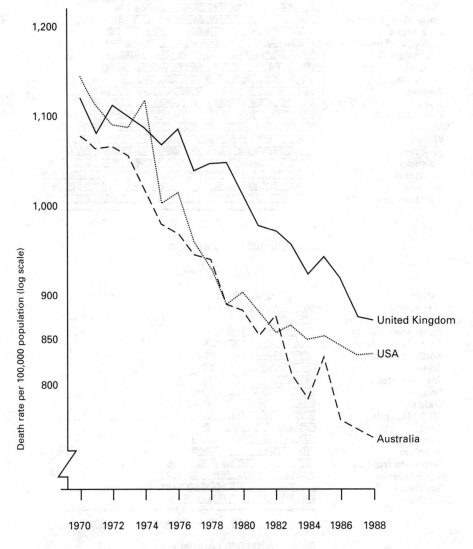

*Rates are calculated using the European Standard Population
Source: WHO[24]

2.1.6   *Geographic variations.*

2.1.6.1 *Variations in the UK*   Standardised death rates for both CHD and stroke show a clear geographic pattern of distribution, with in general, higher rates in the northern regions of England, and in Scotland and Northern Ireland (see Figures 2.8a to 2.8d).

Figure 2.8a Death rates* for coronary heart disease by region of United Kingdom, 1990

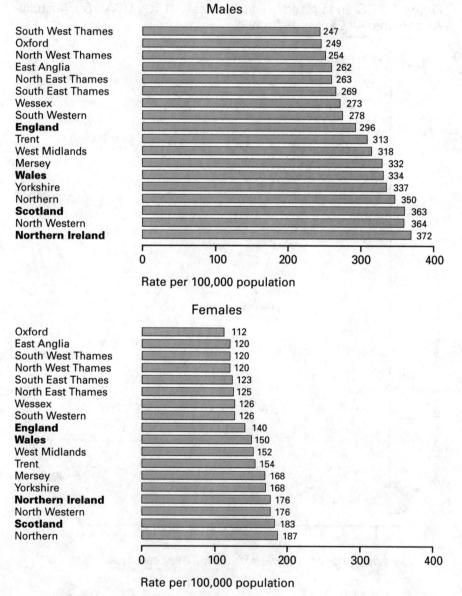

Males

Region	Rate
South West Thames	247
Oxford	249
North West Thames	254
East Anglia	262
North East Thames	263
South East Thames	269
Wessex	273
South Western	278
England	296
Trent	313
West Midlands	318
Mersey	332
Wales	334
Yorkshire	337
Northern	350
Scotland	363
North Western	364
Northern Ireland	372

Rate per 100,000 population

Females

Region	Rate
Oxford	112
East Anglia	120
South West Thames	120
North West Thames	120
South East Thames	123
North East Thames	125
Wessex	126
South Western	126
England	140
Wales	150
West Midlands	152
Trent	154
Mersey	168
Yorkshire	168
Northern Ireland	176
North Western	176
Scotland	183
Northern	187

Rate per 100,000 population

*Rates calculated using the European Standard Population

Source: OPCS[21]; Registrar General's Offices of Scotland and N. Ireland

Figure 2.8b Death rates* for stroke by region of England with Wales, Northern Ireland and Scotland, 1990

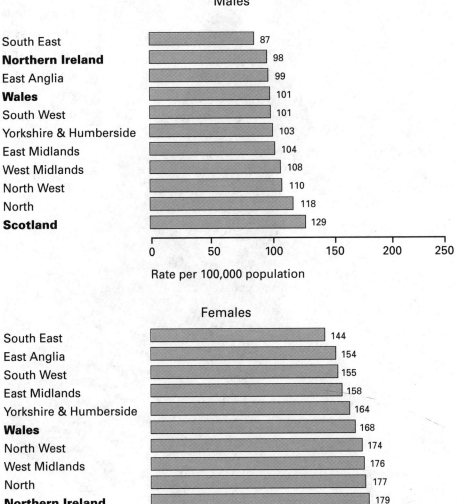

Males

Region	Rate
South East	87
Northern Ireland	98
East Anglia	99
Wales	101
South West	101
Yorkshire & Humberside	103
East Midlands	104
West Midlands	108
North West	110
North	118
Scotland	129

Rate per 100,000 population

Females

Region	Rate
South East	144
East Anglia	154
South West	155
East Midlands	158
Yorkshire & Humberside	164
Wales	168
North West	174
West Midlands	176
North	177
Northern Ireland	179
Scotland	206

Rate per 100,000 population

*Rates calculated using the European Standard Population

Source: OPCS[21]

49

Figure 2.8c Mortality rates from coronary heart disease by District Health Authorities in persons aged 65–74, 1987–1991.

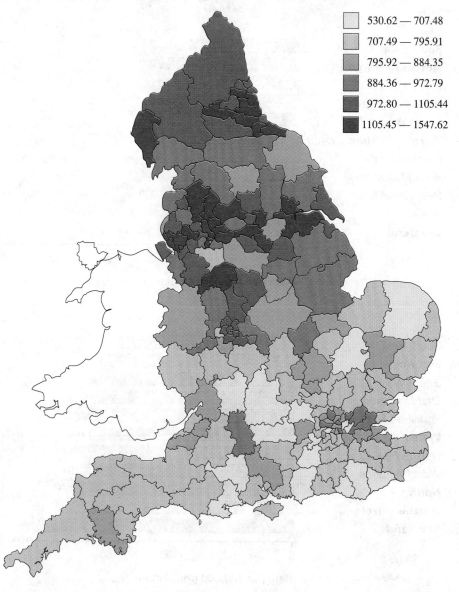

530.62 — 707.48
707.49 — 795.91
795.92 — 884.35
884.36 — 972.79
972.80 — 1105.44
1105.45 — 1547.62

Source: OPCS[21]

Figure 2.8d Mortality rates from stroke by District Health Authorities in persons aged 65–74, 1987–1991

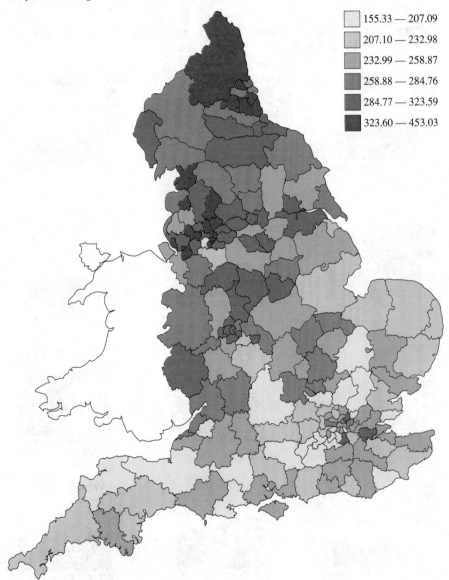

	155.33 — 207.09
	207.10 — 232.98
	232.99 — 258.87
	258.88 — 284.76
	284.77 — 323.59
	323.60 — 453.03

Source: OPCS[21]

2.1.6.2 *International variations in mortality* Comparison of trends in mortality rates from CHD for the 12 European Community (EC) countries show marked differences (see Figure 2.9). In 1988 the CHD mortality rate for all people in Ireland was 260 per 100,000 population, nearly four times the rate in France (67) and also much higher than rates in Mediterranean countries. In some countries, such as Belgium and the Netherlands, there has been a decline in mortality since 1970, whilst in Greece, there has been an increase. Although the rate for the United Kingdom is declining, in 1984 it was the second highest rate in the EC after Ireland.

Figure 2.9 Coronary heart disease mortality in the European Community 1970–1989

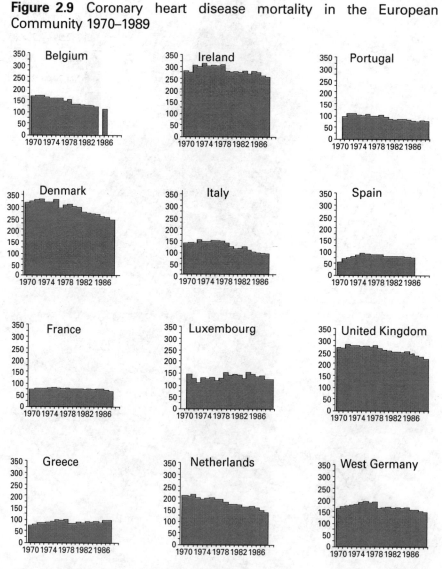

Standardised death rates per 100,000 population for All Persons

Source: WHO[24]

2.1.6.3 Mortality rates for stroke also differ widely between EC Member States but with different patterns from CHD (see Figure 2.10). Rates are declining in most Member States. Portugal had the highest rate in 1988, 210 per 100,000 population, over three times that of France which at 62 per 100,000 population was the lowest. Portugal's high levels of stroke mortality contrast with the lower levels of mortality from CHD compared with most other member states. Conversely the high levels of CHD mortality in Ireland and Denmark contrast with comparatively low levels of stroke mortality. The stroke mortality rate for the United Kingdom declined steadily from 1970 to a level in 1984 which was at the lower end of the range for Member States.

Figure 2.10 Stroke mortality in the European Community 1970–1989

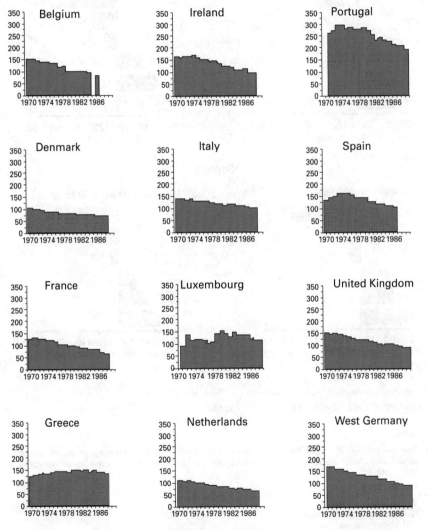

Standardised death rates per 100,000 population for All Persons

Source: WHO[24]

2.1.7 *Social class variations* Figure 2.11 shows that there are social class variations for both CHD and stroke in Great Britain. The pattern of variation is similar for both diseases and for both sexes. There is a consistent trend of increasing mortality, rising from lower than expected in social class I to higher than expected for social class V.

Figure 2.11 Variations in mortality by social class and sex, Great Britain 1979–1983

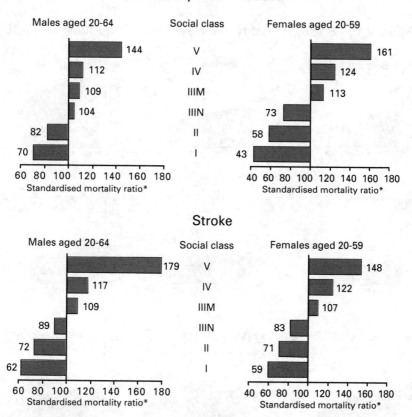

Coronary Heart Disease

Males aged 20-64 — Social class — Females aged 20-59

Social class	Males	Females
V	144	161
IV	112	124
IIIM	109	113
IIIN	104	73
II	82	58
I	70	43

Standardised mortality ratio*

Stroke

Males aged 20-64 — Social class — Females aged 20-59

Social class	Males	Females
V	179	148
IV	117	122
IIIM	109	107
IIIN	89	83
II	72	71
I	62	59

Standardised mortality ratio*

*All values of standardised mortality ratios are significant at the 1% level.

Source: OPCS[25] (CHD ICD 410:414 & Stroke ICD 430:438)

Footnotes

(1) The Standardised Mortality Ratio is an index which adjusts for differences in age structure. Values above 100 indicate higher mortality than the England and Wales average; values below 100 indicate lower mortality.

(2) Social Classes:

V   Unskilled occupations
IV   Partly skilled occupations
IIIM Skilled manual occupations
IIIN Skilled non-manual occupations
II   Intermediate occupations
I   Professional etc occupations

54

2.1.8 *Variations by ethnic origin* Figure 2.12 shows variations in CHD and stroke mortality in England and Wales by ethnic origin as assessed by country of birth. Mortality from CHD amongst males aged 20–69 born in the Indian sub-continent is 36% higher than among the population of England and Wales as a whole and amongst females aged 20–69 it is 46% higher. For those born in the Caribbean commonwealth CHD mortality rates are lower than the population as a whole. This contrasts with higher stroke mortality than the population as a whole amongst both males and females born in the Caribbean commonwealth. For those born in the Indian sub-continent and the African commonwealth stroke

Figure 2.12 Variations in deaths from coronary heart disease and stroke by sex and ethnic origin 1979–1983

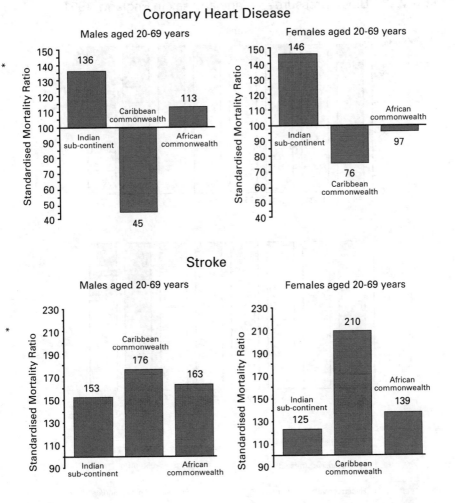

*The Standardised Mortality Ratio is an index which adjusts for differences in age structure. Values above 100 indicate higher mortality than the England and Wales average; values below 100 indicate lower mortality.

Source: Balarajan, 1991[26]

55

mortality rates are also higher than the England and Wales average although not as high as for those from the Caribbean. Those born in the African common-wealth consist of two main groups: East African Asians and Africans. Not surprisingly, the ratios for this group as a whole are intermediate between those for the Indian sub-continent and Caribbean commonwealth groups.

2.2 Cardiovascular risk factors

2.2.1 Blood pressure

In 1991 13% of men were classified as hypertensive (untreated) and 4% as hypertensive (treated)[27] (Figure 2.13). The corresponding figures for women were 11% and 6%, respectively. Men living in the North had a slightly higher mean systolic pressure than those living in the other regions.

Figure 2.13 Blood pressure – by age and sex in England, 1991

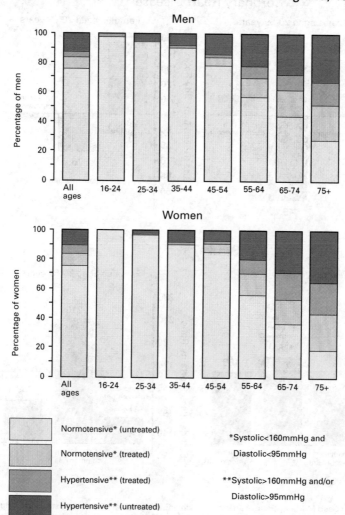

Percentages may not add up to 100, due to rounding

Source: The Health Survey for England, (1991) White *et al*, 1993[27]

56

2.2.2 *Serum cholesterol* Figure 2.14 shows average serum cholesterol in Great Britain by sex and age. In 1986/87 the mean serum total cholesterol concentration was 5.8 mmol/l for both sexes, and increased with age. Amongst subjects in the 1991 Health Survey for England who were aged 19–64, and who were not taking lipid lowering drugs, the mean serum cholesterol concentration

Figure 2.14 Total cholesterol by age and sex, Great Britain, 1986–1987

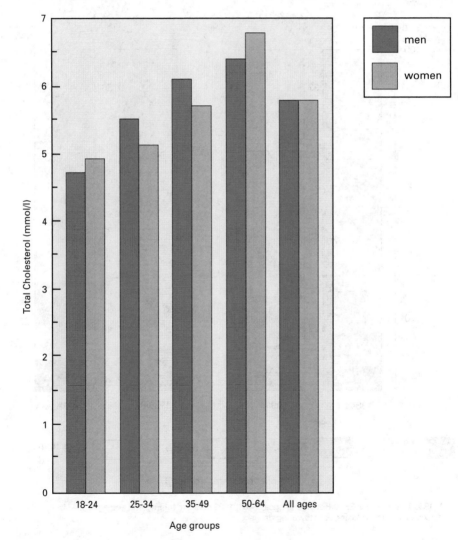

Source: The Dietary and Nutritional Survey of British Adults, (1986/87) Gregory *et al*, 1990[4]

was 5.7 mmol/l for both sexes[27]. Figure 2.15 shows that in 1986/87 32% of males had serum cholesterol levels in the desirable range of less than 5.2 mmol/l compared to 36% for females (see also Appendix A). In 1991 31% and 30% of men and women, respectively, had levels of less than 5.2 mmol/l. There is little regional variation in mean cholesterol levels.

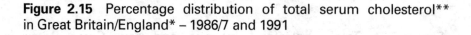

Figure 2.15 Percentage distribution of total serum cholesterol** in Great Britain/England* – 1986/7 and 1991

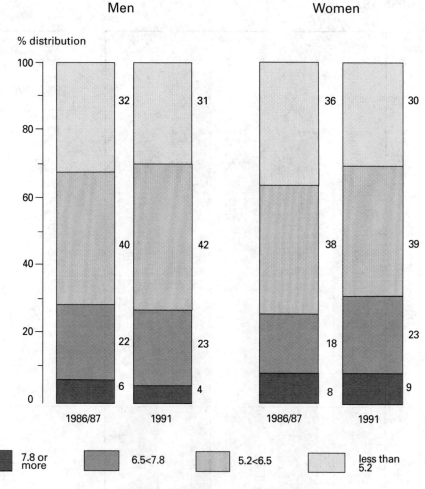

* 1986/7 data are for Great Britain and ages 18–64; 1991 data are for England and ages 18–74
** Excludes persons taking lipid lowering drugs

Sources:
The Dietary and Nutritional Survey of British Adults, (1986/7) Gregory *et al*, 1990[4]
The Health Survey for England, (1991) White *et al*, 1993[27]

2.2.3 *Obesity* Figure 2.16 shows the distribution of body mass index (BMI) by sex from surveys in Great Britain. In 1986/87, 12% of women and 8% of men were obese, with BMI in excess of 30, compared to 8% and 6% respectively in 1980. By 1991 these figures had increased to 15% and 13% respectively.

Figure 2.16 Body mass index in men and women in Great Britain/England* in 1980, 1986/7 and 1991 – aged 16 to 64 years

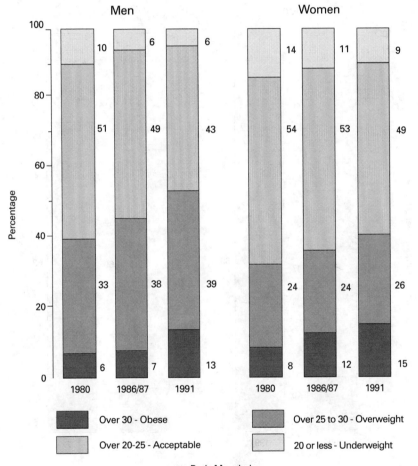

Body Mass Index
Percentages may not add up to 100 due to rounding

* 1980 data are for Great Britain, other data are for England

Sources:
The Heights and Weights of Adults in Great Britain, (1980) OPCS, 1984[28]
The Dietary and Nutritional Survey of British Adults, (1986/7) Gregory *et al*, 1990[4]
The Health Survey for England, (1991) White *et al*, 1993[27]

2.2.4   *Physical activity*   Figure 2.17 compares the findings from the 1990 Allied Dunbar National Fitness Survey[29] with those of the 1991 Health Survey for England[27]. A higher proportion of men than women reported vigorous activity in both surveys.

Figure 2.17   Physical activity in men and women in England in 1990 and 1991 – aged 16 to 74 years

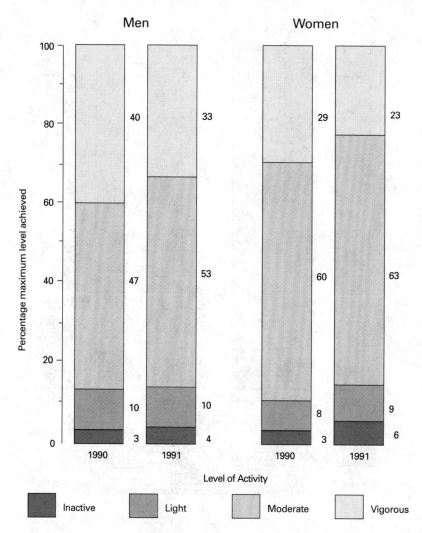

Sources:
National Fitness Survey, Allied Dunbar (1990), 1992[29]
The Health Survey for England, (1991) White *et al*, 1993[27]

2.2.5 *Alcohol* The percentage of the population drinking more than the recommended sensible limits (21 units per week for males and 14 units for females) is 27% of males and 11% for females (see Figure 2.18).

Figure 2.18 Distribution of drinkers aged 18 and over by sex and consumption category, Great Britain 1990

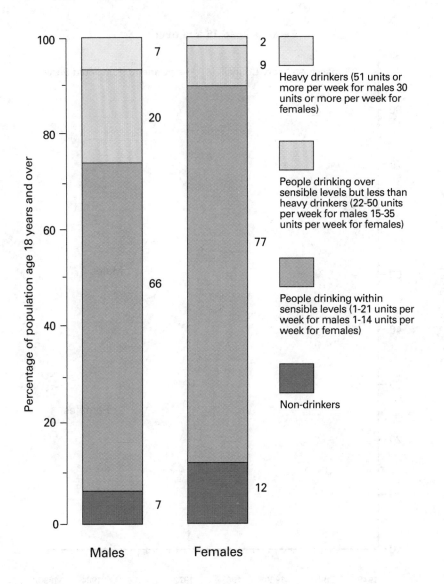

Heavy drinkers (51 units or more per week for males 30 units or more per week for females)

People drinking over sensible levels but less than heavy drinkers (22-50 units per week for males 15-35 units per week for females)

People drinking within sensible levels (1-21 units per week for males 1-14 units per week for females)

Non-drinkers

Source: OPCS General Household Survey, 1990[30]

2.2.6 *Cigarette smoking* The percentage of cigarette smokers in the population continues to decline in Great Britain (Figure 2.19). The decline for females has not been as steep as that for males. The gap between males and females has narrowed from 12 percentage points in 1972 to 2 percentage points in 1990,

Figure 2.19 Percentage of cigarette smokers in the population, Great Britain, 1948–1990

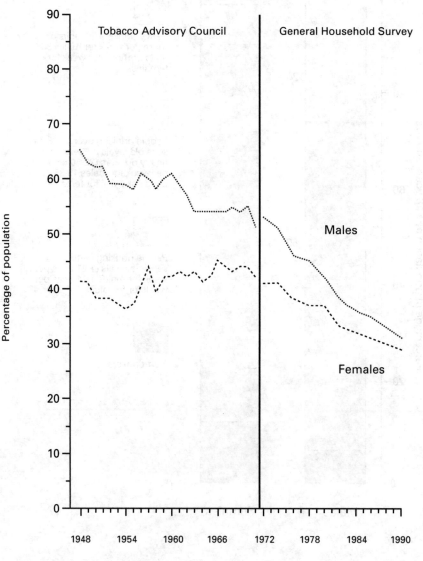

Persons aged 16 and over

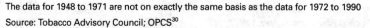
The data for 1948 to 1971 are not on exactly the same basis as the data for 1972 to 1990

Source: Tobacco Advisory Council; OPCS[30]

when 31% of males and 29% of females were smokers. Figure 2.20 shows trends by sex and age group. The downward trend has shown recent signs of levelling off or beginning to reverse in the younger age groups. Figure 2.21 shows that

Figure 2.20 Percentage of cigarette smokers in the population by sex and age, Great Britain 1972–90

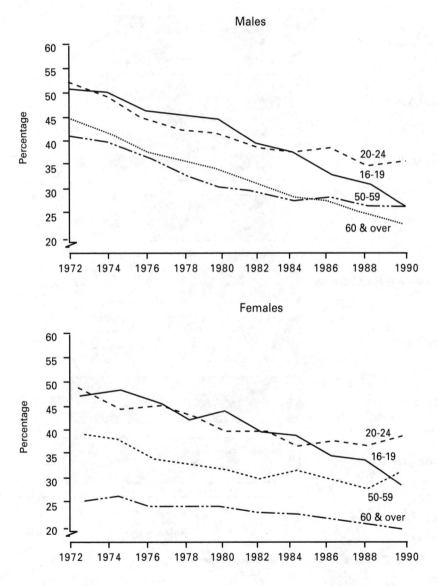

Source: OPCS[30]

smoking prevalence tends to be higher in the northern regions. Although data on cigarette smoking and alcohol consumption are available from the Health Survey for England, we have used the data from the General Household Survey because of its larger sample size.

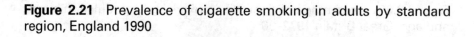

Figure 2.21 Prevalence of cigarette smoking in adults by standard region, England 1990

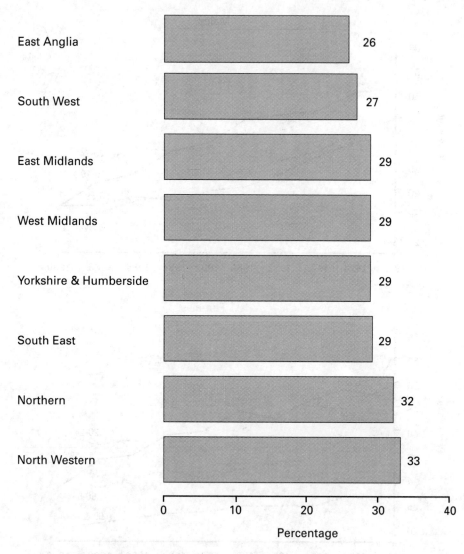

Source: OPCS General Household Survey (unpublished data)

2.2.7 *International comparisons in risk factors* Information on 4 major risk factors in 7 European countries in the MONICA study is shown in Figures 2.22–2.25[24]. These data are from selected towns and are not intended to be representative of the whole population. Except for systolic blood pressure, the variations in levels of the other risk factors across these countries is not great. Denmark has a relatively high death rate for CHD and the highest levels of raised

Figure 2.22 Systolic blood pressure (mmHg) distribution. Age-standardised proportions by selected categories in MONICA populations

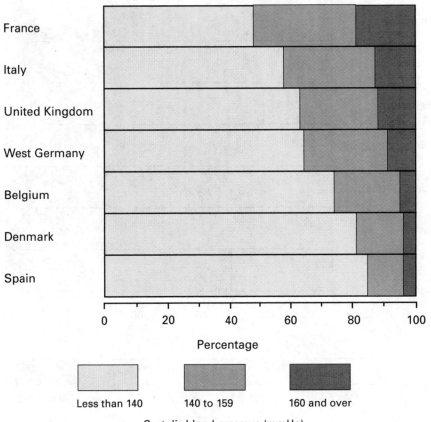

Males aged 35-64 years

Percentage

Systolic blood pressure (mmHg)

Less than 140   140 to 159   160 and over

*Values for countries with more than one MONICA centre are based on weighted averages of the individual centre values
France: Bas-Rhin and Lille
Italy: Area Latina, Friuli and Area Brianza
United Kingdom: Glasgow and Belfast
West Germany: Augsburg (rural), Augsburg (urban), Bremen and Rhein-Necker Region
Belgium: Charleroi, Ghent and Luxembourg

Source: WHO[24]

blood cholesterol among the 7 countries, but scores lowest with Spain for the other risk factors. Denmark has the highest consumption of butter plus margarine, and is next to the lowest for consumption of fruit and vegetables (Figure 2.43). Though France has at least average levels of systolic blood pressure, plasma cholesterol, body mass index and smoking, it has the lowest mortality from cardiovascular disease (Figures 2.9 and 2.10).

Figure 2.23 Total cholesterol (mmol/l) distribution age-standardised proportions by selected categories in MONICA populations

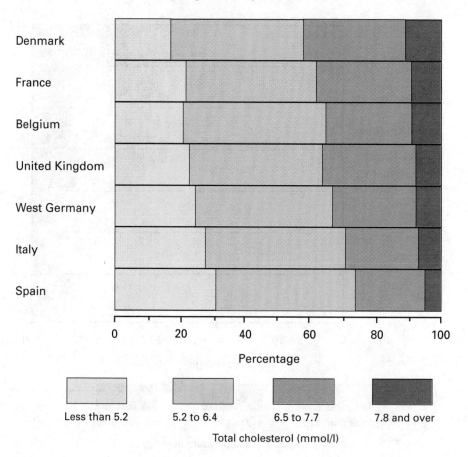

Males aged 35-64 years

*Values for countries with more than one MONICA centre are based on weighted averages of the individual centre values
France: Lille and Haute-Garonne
Belgium: Charleroi and Ghent
West Germany: Augsburg (rural), Augsburg (urban), Bremen and Rhein-Necker Region
United Kingdom: Glasgow and Belfast
Italy: Area Latina, Friuli and Area Brianza
Source: WHO[24]

Figure 2.24 Body mass index (kg/m^2) distribution. Age-standardised proportions by selected categories in MONICA populations

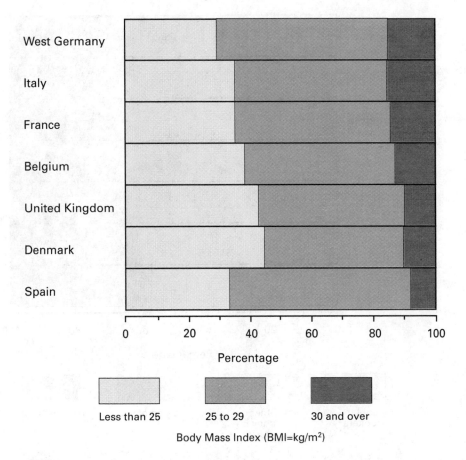

Males aged 35-64 years

Percentage

Less than 25   25 to 29   30 and over

Body Mass Index (BMI=kg/m^2)

*Values for countries with more than one MONICA centre are based on weighted averages of the individual centre values
West Germany: Augsburg (rural), Augsburg (urban), Bremen and Rhein-Necker Region
Italy: Area Latina, Friuli and Area Brianza
France: Bas-Rhin, Lille and Haute-Garonne
Belgium: Charleroi, Ghent and Luxembourg Province
United Kingdom: Glasgow and Belfast

Source: WHO[24]

67

Figure 2.25 Smoking distribution. Age-standardised proportions by selected categories in MONICA populations

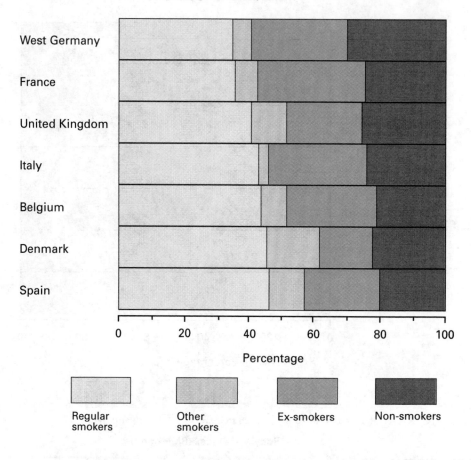

Males aged 35-64 years

Percentage

Regular smokers | Other smokers | Ex-smokers | Non-smokers

*Values for countries with more than one MONICA centre are based on weighted averages of the individual centre values
West Germany: Augsburg (rural), Augsburg (urban), Bremen and Rhein-Necker Region
France: Bas-Rhin, Lille and Haute-Garonne
United Kingdom: Glasgow and Belfast
Italy: Area Latina, Friuli and Area Brianza
Belgium: Charleroi, Ghent and Luxembourg Province

Source: WHO[24]

2.3 The British diet

2.3.1 *Sources of information* Information can be obtained from three sources: the National Food Survey (NFS) conducted by the Ministry of Agriculture, Fisheries and Food (MAFF)[31]; the Dietary and Nutritional Survey of British Adults, conducted by OPCS for MAFF and DH in 1986/7[4]; and OECD Food Consumption Statistics[32].

2.3.1.1 *The National Food Survey* The continuous NFS is an inquiry into the amounts and cost of foods obtained by private households in Britain and of its nutrient content. Over 7000 households per year participate in this nationally representative survey which has been ongoing since 1940. The householder keeps a seven day record of the description, quantity, and cost of all food entering the home for human consumption. Information on confectionery, alcoholic and soft drinks and meals purchased outside the home has also been collected since January 1992. The NFS provides information on long-term trends in national food and nutrient intakes and variations in intake by groups of the population (e.g. by regional and socio-economic characteristics). It cannot, however, provide information about the nutrient intake of individuals within the population.

2.3.1.2 *The Dietary and Nutritional Survey of British Adults* The 1986/87 Dietary and Nutritional Survey of British Adults[4] provides detailed nutrient and food intake data for approximately 2200 individuals aged 16–64 years and provides valuable information on the detailed composition of the diets of individuals throughout Britain. As well as measuring dietary intakes by means of 7-day weighed records, measurements of height, weight and blood pressure were taken, and blood and urine were analyzed for various nutritional parameters. This successful survey has now been expanded to comprise a programme of National Diet and Nutrition Surveys, combining dietary assessments with anthropometry, measures of nutritional status and other relevant physiological variables. The programme is intended to cover all ages beyond infancy in four age groups (children aged 1½ - 4½ years, schoolchildren, adults aged 16–64 years and adults aged 65 years and over) in a rolling programme over about a decade. Currently data from the survey of children aged 1½ to 4½ years are being analyzed (see 7.5) and fieldwork is being planned for a survey of adults aged 65 years and over.

2.3.1.3 *OECD Food Consumption Statistics* These are estimates of the national food supplies of the OECD countries, and record the proportion of the agricultural production entering the human food chain after the deduction of food exports plus the addition of food imports. This information is collected in a consistent way for each country but substantially over-estimates the amount of food and nutrients actually eaten.

2.3.2 Trends in the British diet 1940–1992

2.3.2.1 The broad pattern of changes in the British diet over the last 50 years can be seen from the National Food Survey and is shown in Figures 2.26 and 2.27. There was a decline in the proportion of food energy derived from carbohydrate, and a corresponding increase in the proportion of energy derived from fat, in the years following the War but the balance of energy from carbohydrate, fat and protein has remained steady over the last 20 years (Figure 2.26). There have, however, been substantial changes in the types and quantities of foods consumed over this period.

2.3.2.2 *Milk*   During the War, successful efforts were made to increase milk consumption, and intake then remained relatively stable at around (390 ml/day) until the mid 1970s. Whole milk consumption fell to around 340 ml/day in 1980 and to 140 ml/day in 1992. Skimmed milks, which were hardly consumed in 1980 were at a consumption level of 140 ml/day in 1992. This trend seems to be continuing and currently about 50 % of the liquid milk market is for skimmed (mainly semi skimmed) milks.

2.3.2.3 *Fats and oils*   Total consumption of fats and oils remained steady at around 50 g/day from the mid 1950s to the early 1970s, but consumption has dropped to around 35 g/day in 1992. The relative importance of individual foods within the fats group has changed, with increased consumption of low fat spreads, polyunsaturated margarines and vegetable oils in place of butter, hard margarines and lard. Butter consumption decreased from around 24 g/day in the late 1950s, to about 16 g/day in 1980, to around 6 g/day in 1992 (Figure 2.28).

2.3.2.4 *Meats*   Consumption of beef, lamb and pork all rose sharply in the mid 1950s, but since then the main change has been a steady decline in lamb and a considerable increase in poultry consumption. Poultry is now more popular than beef (33 g/day vs. 20 g/day). Among meat products, the most important change has been the increasing popularity of convenience products and more recently, items such as paté.

Figure 2.26   Trends in proportion of daily energy intake derived from carbohydrate, fat and protein

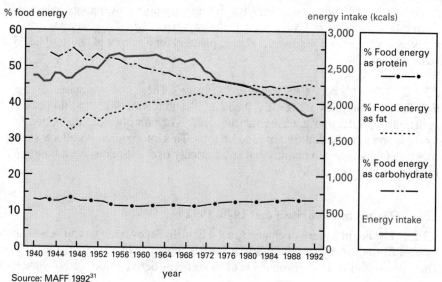

Source: MAFF 1992[31]

Figure 2.27 Consumption of selected foods

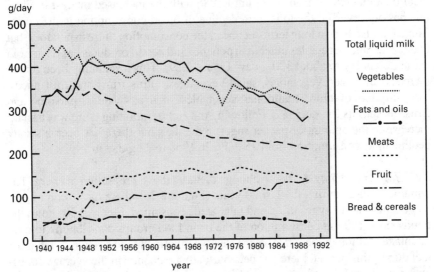

g/day

Total liquid milk

Vegetables

Fats and oils

Meats

Fruit

Bread & cereals

year

Source: MAFF 1992[31]

2.3.2.5 *Fish* Total fish consumption has fallen from around 27g/day in 1950 to 20g/day in 1990 of which 7g was oily fish. However fish consumption is highly skewed and the Dietary and Nutritional Survey of British Adults showed that consumers of oily fish had intakes of around 19g/day.

2.3.2.6 *Bread, vegetables and fruit* Bread consumption has fallen consistently since 1940 from around 250 g/day to 110 g/day. The consumption of National Wheatmeal Bread, introduced during the second world war, declined rapidly

Figure 2.28 Trends in consumption of fats

g/day

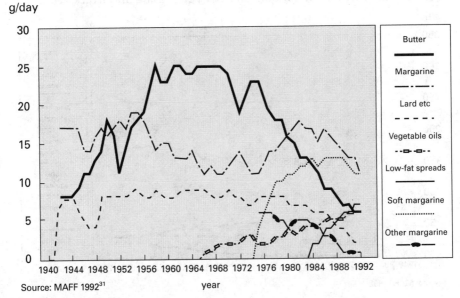

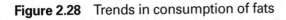

Butter

Margarine

Lard etc

Vegetable oils

Low-fat spreads

Soft margarine

Other margarine

year

Source: MAFF 1992[31]

after white bread was reintroduced in 1955. Although consumption of whole-meal bread increased from 1978 until 1986 with the increased interest in fibre, this has not reversed the long term decline of bread consumption in the home. There has also been a long term decline in the consumption of fresh potatoes, but that of fruit and vegetables other than potatoes and potato products has risen from about 200 g/day to about 300 g/day (Figure 2.29). This has mainly been due to increases in frozen vegetables, salad vegetables, citrus fruits and fruit juices. Consumption of more traditional vegetables such as swedes, parsnips and Brussels sprouts has declined. Following the end of rationing there was a sharp increase in the amount of packet sugar in the diet, but there has been a steady decline in its consumption from 75 g/day in 1958 to 22 g/day in 1992.

2.3.2.7 *Fats and fatty acids*   Although dietary fat as a proportion of energy has remained steady during the last 20 years (Figure 2.26), there have been important changes in the types of fat and fatty acids consumed. Figure 2.30 shows the trends since 1955 in consumption of the main food groups contributing to total fat intake. Although there has been a steady reduction in the amount of fat in the diet during this period, there has been virtually no change in the average contribution made by fat to energy derived from food (Figure 2.26). This is because the amount of carbohydrate and the amount of energy in the diet have also decreased. NFS data for 1992 shows that fat still provides 41–42% of food energy.

2.3.2.8 Figure 2.31 shows the trends since 1959 in the average proportion of food energy derived from the main fatty acids and the ratio of polyunsaturated to saturated fatty acids in the diet (P/S ratio). The intake of saturated fatty acids started to fall in the early 1970s, and since 1980, intake of saturated fatty acids has declined from 19% of food energy to 16% of food energy in 1992 (Figure 2.31). During this time there has been a corresponding increase in poly-unsaturated fatty acids, from 5% in 1980 to 7% in 1992. These changes have

Figure 2.29   Trends in consumption of vegetables and fruit

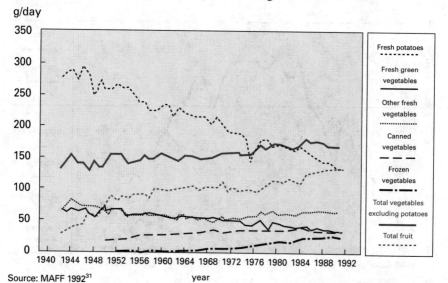

Source: MAFF 1992[31]

Figure 2.30 Contribution made by food groups to fat consumption

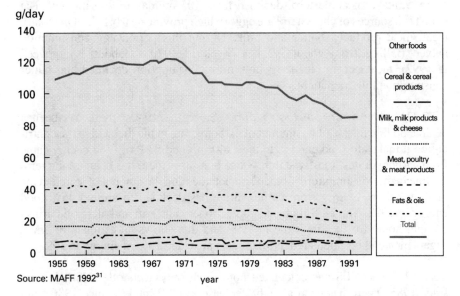

Source: MAFF 1992[31]

resulted in a rise in the P/S ratio from around 0.2 to 0.4. During this time, intake of monounsaturated fatty acids has remained fairly constant at around 15 % of food energy.

2.3.2.9   There has been increasing interest in the consumption of trans fatty acids in recent years, and current intake from the NFS has been estimated at around 2% of food energy.

Figure 2.31 Trends in intake of fatty acids

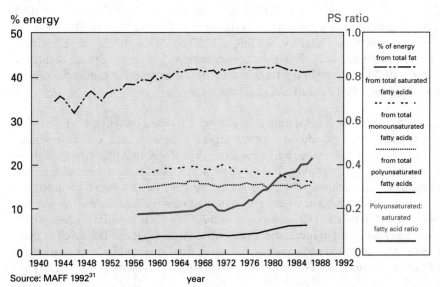

Source: MAFF 1992[31]

2.3.2.10   *Dietary cholesterol*   Between 1970/75 and 1992 the national average intake of cholesterol declined from 405 mg/day to 245 mg/day. The main food sources of cholesterol are eggs (which provide nearly half of the total), meat, meat products, butter and milk. During this period egg consumption halved (falling from about 2.2 eggs/week in 1970 to about 1 egg/week in 1992), meat became leaner, whole milk consumption declined and butter consumption fell dramatically.

2.3.2.11 *Carbohydrates, including fibre*   Since the 1940s, there has been a decline both in the absolute amount of carbohydrate in the diet and in the contribution it makes to food energy. In the 1940s around 53% of food energy came from carbohydrates, mostly starch. Since that time, there has been a long term decline in the consumption of bread and potatoes and the amount of starch in the diet has fallen. Energy from carbohydrate has declined to around 45% food energy in 1992. The NFS included confectionery and soft and alcoholic drinks brought home for the first time in 1992 and this allows an estimate of NME sugars intake to be calculated. NME sugars provided 13% of energy in 1992.

2.3.2.12   The NFS has calculated non-starch polysaccharide (NSP) intakes since 1985. There has been a slight decrease in NSP intakes since 1986 from 13 g/day in 1986 to 12 g/day in 1992. About 50% of NSP is provided by cereal products such as bread and 50% by fruit and vegetables.

2.3.2.13   *Vitamin C*   Absolute intake of vitamin C has remained relatively constant at around 50–60 mg/day since the 1950s. However, since energy intakes have fallen considerably over this period, the concentration of vitamin C in the diet has increased (from 20 mg/1000 kcal in the 1950s to 27 mg/1000 kcal in 1992). Approximately 80 % of dietary vitamin C is provided by fruits and vegetables, and until the mid 1980s potatoes were the main source. Since that time, fruit juices have become the main source due to increased consumption.

2.3.2.14   *β-carotene*   The NFS has calculated intakes of β-carotene since 1969, when the diet contained 2110 μg/day. During the 1980s intake of β-carotene increased slightly, but fell to 1750 μg/day in 1992. There has been very little change since 1969 in the concentration of β-carotene in the diet (from 820 μg /1000 kcal to 940 μg/1000 kcal in 1992). Around 70 % of β-carotene in the diet is provided by fruit and vegetables, the main source being carrots.

2.3.2.15   *Vitamin E*   Vitamin E intake was first measured in the NFS in 1979 where intake was calculated to be 8.3 mg/day. Tea was calculated as providing 2.2 mg/day of total intake, but it has since been suggested that vitamin E from this source is not available. Thus, 6.1 mg/day came from other sources. This compares with an intake of 8.2 mg/day during 1992 (tea no longer included as a source of vitamin E). The main contributors to vitamin E intake are oils and fats (47% of total intake in 1992 compared with 26% of the total in 1979). Since 1979 there has been a rapid increase in the consumption of fats and oils rich in poly-unsaturated fatty acids, and thus in vitamin E. Sunflower oil is the richest source of the most potent form of vitamin E, RRR alpha-tocopherol. Other significant sources of vitamin E in the British diet are vegetables (15% total intake) and cereals (13% total intake).

2.3.3   The diets of British adults

2.3.3.1 The Dietary and Nutritional Survey of British Adults (the 'Adults Survey') which was carried out during 1986/87[4], measured the diets of individual adults aged 16–64 years. The dietary pattern observed for adults during 1986/87 was broadly similar to the national average diet seen from the NFS.

2.3.3.2 *Fats and fatty acids*   The average daily intake of fat was 102 g for men and 74 g for women. This corresponds to around 40% of food energy in both cases (due to the lower energy intakes of women). Because men derived a greater proportion of their total energy from alcohol than women (6.9% *vs*. 2.8%) women obtained a greater proportion of their total energy from fat than men. 12% of men and 15% of women had fat intakes of less than 35% food energy. Women obtained a slightly higher proportion of total (and food) energy from saturated fatty acids than men. Energy from saturated fatty acids was also greater for those aged 50–64 years compared with the younger age groups (Tables 2.1 and 2.2). Energy intakes from monounsaturated, polyunsaturated and trans fatty acids were similar for both sexes.

2.3.3.3. Average intake of n-6 polyunsaturates was 13.8 g/day (5.1% total energy) and 9.6 g/day (5.1% total energy) for men and women respectively. Individuals aged 50–64 years had a lower intake of n-6 polyunsaturates, both in men and women. The average daily intake of n-3 polyunsaturates was much lower at 1.9 g (0.7% total energy) for men and 1.3 g (0.7% total energy) for women. Intake of n-3 polyunsaturates was significantly lower in older men (50–64 years), but less markedly lower in the oldest group of women. Population average intakes of longer chain n-3 polyunsaturates, eg EPA and DHA from oily fish were about 0.1g/day for men and women. Intakes in consumers of oily fish were higher at 0.3g/day for men and 0.2g/day for women.

2.3.3.4 The average P/S ratio was higher for men than women (0.40 *vs*. 0.38). Those over 50 years had a lower average P/S ratio than those under 50 years. Trans fatty acid intake was, on average, 5.6 g/day (2.0% total energy) for men and 4.0 g/day (2.1% total energy) for women.

2.3.3.5 *Dietary cholesterol*   Intake of cholesterol was about 40 % higher in men than in women (390 mg/day *vs*. 280 mg/day). Cholesterol intake increased with age. For both sexes those aged 50–64 years had significantly higher intakes than the youngest age group (16–24 years), in spite of the lower total energy intakes of the older group.

2.3.3.6 *Carbohydrates including dietary fibre*   Men had an average carbohydrate intake of 272 g/day (41.6% total energy) compared with 193 g/day (43% total energy) for women. Total carbohydrate intakes were markedly lower for those aged 50–64 years compared with those aged 16–24 years. The percentage

Table 2.1 *Intake of selected nutrients by sex – Adults aged 16-64 years*

	Men	% total energy	Women	% total energy
total energy (kcal)	2450		1680	
fat (g)	102	37.6	74	39.2
saturates (g)	42	15.4	31	16.5
monounsaturates (g)	31	11.6	22	11.8
n-3 polyunsaturates (g)	1.9	0.7	1.3	0.7
n-6 polyunsaturates (g)	13.8	5.1	9.6	5.1
trans fatty acids (g)	5.6	2.0	4.0	2.1
P/S ratio	0.40		0.38	
cholesterol (mg)	390		280	
carbohydrate (g)	272	41.6	193	43.0
starch (g)	156	23.9	106	23.7
sugars (g)	115	17.6	86	19.2
alcohol (g)	25	6.9	6.9	2.8
fibre (g)	24.9		18.6	

Source: Dietary & Nutritional Survey of British Adults, Gregory *et al* 1990[4]

Table 2.2 *Intake of selected nutrients by age and sex – Adults aged 16–64 years*

Men	Age 16–24	25–34	35–49	50–64	All 16–64
Total energy (kcal)	2460	2440	2500	2380	2450
% total energy from:					
fat	37.9	37.9	37.1	37.6	37.6
saturates	15.2	15.3	15.1	16.1	15.4
monosaturates	11.9	11.8	11.3	11.3	11.6
n-6 polyunsaturates	5.2	5.2	5.2	4.6	5.1
n-3 polyunsaturates	0.7	0.7	0.7	0.7	0.7
trans fatty acids	2.1	2.0	2.1	2.0	2.0
carbohydrate	42.9	40.9	41.5	41.4	41.6
starch	25.2	23.5	23.7	23.2	23.9
sugars	17.4	17.2	17.6	18.0	17.6
alcohol (total sample)	5.9	7.3	7.6	6.4	6.9
alcohol (consumers only)	8.7	8.7	9.1	8.1	8.7
P/S ratio	0.41	0.43	0.42	0.35	0.40
cholesterol (mg)	362	383	398	407	390
fibre (g)	23.9	24.5	25.8	24.8	24.9

Women	Age 16–24	25–34	35–49	50–64	All 16–64
Total energy (kcal)	1700	1670	1730	1610	1680
% total energy from:					
fat	38.7	39.4	39.0	39.5	39.2
saturates	16.0	16.4	16.4	17.1	16.5
monosaturates	12.0	12.0	11.8	11.7	11.8
n-6 polyunsaturates	5.2	5.3	5.1	4.9	5.1
n-3 polyunsaturates	0.8	0.7	0.7	0.7	0.7
trans fatty acids	2.1	2.1	2.1	2.1	2.1
carbohydrate	44.9	43.0	42.5	42.3	43.0
starch	24.5	23.8	23.2	23.8	23.7
sugars	20.3	19.1	19.3	18.4	19.2
alcohol (total sample)	2.5	3.1	3.2	2.2	2.8
alcohol (consumers only)	4.7	4.3	4.6	3.5	4.3
P/S ratio	0.40	0.39	0.38	0.35	0.38
cholesterol (mg)	247	264	295	294	280
fibre (g)	17.4	18.2	18.9	19.3	18.6

Source: Dietary & Nutritional Survey of British Adults, Gregory *et al* 1990[4]

of total energy derived from carbohydrate generally decreased with age, particularly among women. Starch intakes were significantly higher in men than in women, and were also higher in the younger age groups. Non-milk extrinsic sugars were not calculated in the Adult Survey but have since been estimated as being around 16% of total energy for men and women[33].

2.3.3.7 Because of their higher food intake in general, average intakes of dietary fibre (measured by the Southgate method) were higher in men than in women (24.9 g/day *vs*. 18.6 g/day). 25% of men and 6% of women had intakes greater than 30 g/day (equivalent to 18 g non-starch polysaccharides/day). About 50% of fibre was provided by cereal products such as bread and 50% by vegetables and fruit.

2.3.3.8 *Vitamins C, E and total carotenes*   There was no significant difference in intakes of vitamin C between men and women, although women had higher intakes from supplements than men. Average intakes from all sources were 75 mg/day in men and 73 mg/day in women. There were no age related differences for men in intakes of vitamin C from all sources, but women aged 16–24 years had intakes markedly lower than the overall average for women (62 mg/day). Vitamin E intakes from all sources, including supplements, were higher in men than in women (11.7 mg/day *vs*. 8.6 mg/day) and supplements were an equally important source in men and women. Carotene intakes were slightly higher in men than in women (2410 μg/day *vs*. 2130 μg/day). Carotene intake was lower in the 16–24 year old group (1890 μg/day in men and 1580 µg/day in women). Fruit and vegetables are the major source of vitamin C and carotenes in the diet, providing around 80% of vitamin C and 70% of β-carotene. The major sources of vitamin E are vegetable oils and the products containing them, eg, polyunsaturated margarines (11%), cereal products (21%), vegetables including fried potatoes (22%) and meat and meat products (11%).

2.3.3.9 *Sodium and potassium*   Average sodium excretion (an accurate measure of sodium intake) was 173 mmol/day in men and 132 mmol/day in women. This is equivalent to 10.2g salt/day (3.9 g sodium) in men and 7.8 g salt/day (3.0 g sodium) in women. Potassium intakes were 3.2 g/day (82 mmol/day) in men and 2.4 g/day (62 mmol/day) in women. The major sources of sodium were bread (22%) and meat products (27%), particularly bacon and ham (11%). The major sources of potassium were vegetables (28%), particularly potatoes (17%), meat and meat products (13%), milk and milk products (14%) and cereal products (14%).

2.3.3.10   *Alcohol*   The average alcohol intake of the total sample was between three and four times higher for men than women (25.0 g/day *vs*. 6.9 g/day). Some 21% of men and 35% of women consumed no alcohol during the survey period, and the distribution of alcohol intake was positively skewed. On average, men obtained 6.9% of total energy from alcohol compared with 2.8% for women. When looking at consumers only, men obtained 8.7% and women 4.3% of total energy from alcohol.

2.3.4 Variations in diet and nutrition according to social class, income group and region

2.3.4.1 *Fat and fatty acids*   The NFS indicates that there are no systematic differences in the proportion of energy derived from fat and saturated fatty acids in different regions or between different income groups of Great Britain. The 1986/87 'Adults' Survey showed a similar pattern. However the P/S ratio was significantly lower in men and women in social classes IV and V compared to those in non-manual classes. The 1992 NFS data show that the difference in P/S ratio between income groups is now small. Since about 1980, the decline in the proportion of energy derived from saturated fatty acids has occurred in all income groups and regions.

2.3.4.2 *Vitamins C and E, and β-carotene*   Figures 2.32–2.37 show the average intakes of vitamins C, E and carotenes by income group and region from the 1992 NFS. Both vitamin C and β-carotene intakes are lower in income groups C and D compared with income groups A and B. Income groups C and D also have a lower intake of fruit and vegetables than income groups A and B. The 'Adults' survey showed a strong effect of social class on intake, with lower intakes in social classes IV and V, and this relationship was particularly marked in women (Figures 2.38–2.40). Regional variations are less but tend towards a lower intake in the North. There are slightly lower intakes of vitamin C in the North and in Scotland and Wales than in the South East. β-carotene intakes are lowest in the North West and Scotland. The consumption of fresh green vegetables and fruit is considerably lower in Scotland than in the South (Figures 2.41–2.42).

Figure 2.32   Vitamin C intake (mg/day) by income group

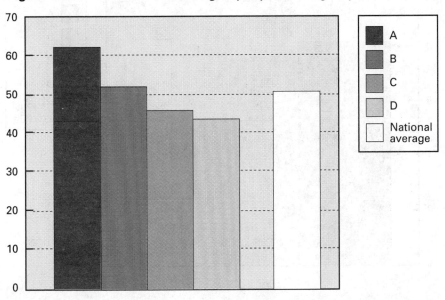

Source: MAFF 1992[31]

Figure 2.33 Vitamin C intake (mg/day) by region

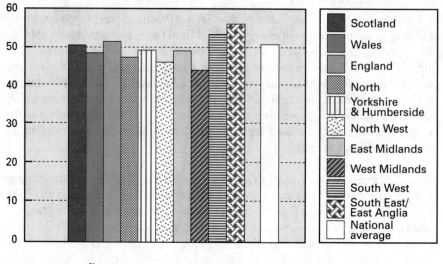

Figure 2.34 Vitamin E intake (mg/day) by income group

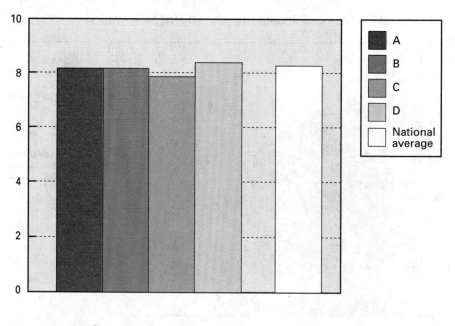

Figure 2.35 Vitamin E intake (mg/day) by region

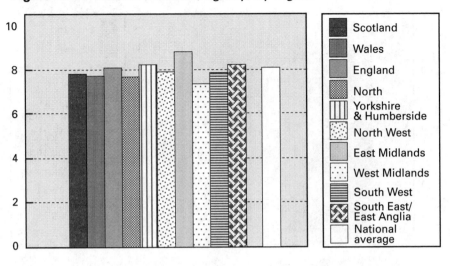

Source: MAFF 1992[31]

Figure 2.36 Beta-carotene intake (µg/day) by income group

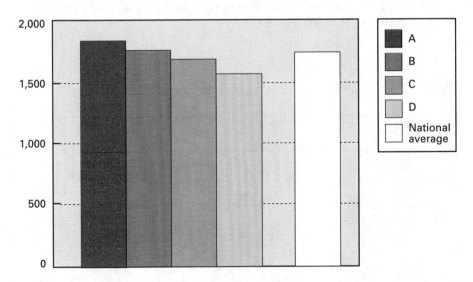

Source: MAFF 1992[31]

Figure 2.37 Beta-carotene intake (µg/day) by region

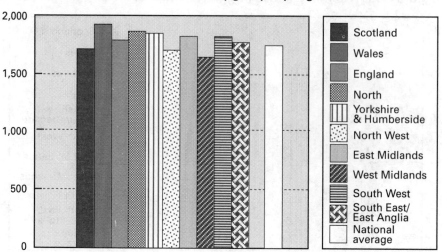

Scotland
Wales
England
North
Yorkshire & Humberside
North West
East Midlands
West Midlands
South West
South East/ East Anglia
National average

Source: MAFF 1992[31]

2.3.4.3 These differences in intakes are reflected in regional and social class differences in plasma levels of *β*-carotene and vitamin E measured in the 'Adults' survey. Men in London and the South East and men in non-manual social classes had significantly higher levels of plasma *β*-carotene and vitamin E than men in the Northern region and men in manual social classes. Women in London and the South East had significantly higher levels of plasma *β*-carotene than women living elsewhere but there was no difference in plasma vitamin E levels. A social class difference was also seen in women with women in non-manual households having significantly higher levels of plasma *β*-carotene and vitamin E than women from manual households.

Figure 2.38 Vitamin C intake (mg/day) by social class and sex

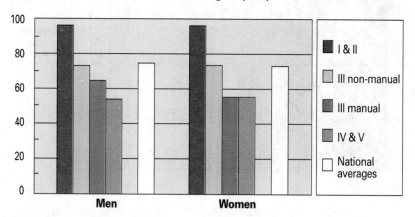

I & II
III non-manual
III manual
IV & V
National averages

Men   Women

Source: Gregory *et al*, 1990[4]

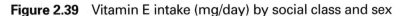

Figure 2.39   Vitamin E intake (mg/day) by social class and sex

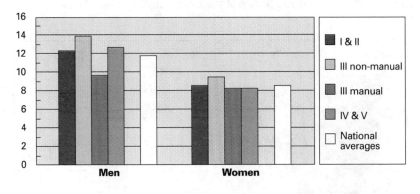

Source: Gregory *et al*, 1990[4]

Figure 2.40   Beta-carotene intake (µg/day) by social class and sex

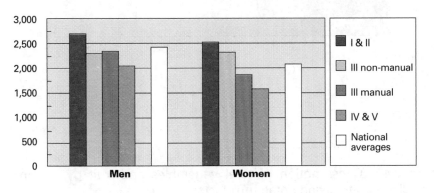

Source: Gregory *et al*, 1990[4]

2.3.4.4 *Alcohol*   The 'Adults' survey showed that among men, those living in Northern England, those in Social Class III manual, and those living without a spouse had higher intakes than others. Among women consumption was higher among those who were employed outside the home.

2.3.5   Cardiovascular disease and diet

2.3.5.1 The secular trend in CHD mortality, particularly the decline since the 1970s, follows a similar course to the trend in the proportion of energy from saturated fatty acids and an inverse trend to that from polyunsaturated fatty acids. The proportion of energy from total fat has been relatively constant over this period, however. The secular trends in CHD mortality and in fruit and vegetable consumption correspond inversely, although there have not been any changes in vitamin C and beta-carotene intakes over this period according to the National Food Survey. The regional and social class differences in CHD mortality in the UK do not correspond to differences in the proportion of energy obtained from

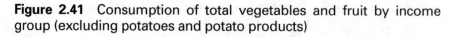

Figure 2.41 Consumption of total vegetables and fruit by income group (excluding potatoes and potato products)

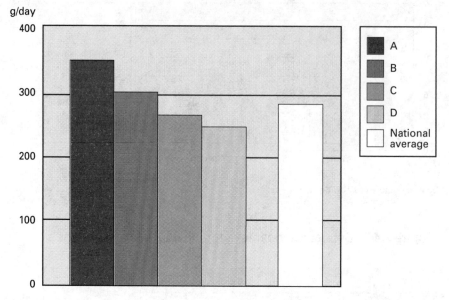

g/day

Legend:
- A
- B
- C
- D
- National average

Source: MAFF 1992[31]

Figure 2.42 Consumption of total vegetables and fruit by region (excluding potatoes and potato products)

g/day

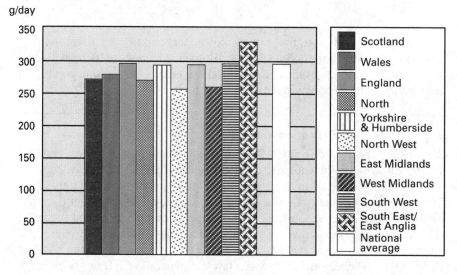

Legend:
- Scotland
- Wales
- England
- North
- Yorkshire & Humberside
- North West
- East Midlands
- West Midlands
- South West
- South East/East Anglia
- National average

Source: MAFF 1992[31]

84

fat or saturated fatty acids (or by differences in plasma cholesterol) but are consistent with the regional and social class differences in intakes of vitamin C and β-carotene and consumption of fruit and vegetables. The relationship between diet and CHD is discussed in Chapter 6 of this report.

2.3.6 The British diet in comparison with other EC countries, the USA and Australia.

(OECD consumption estimates based on food supply statistics.)

2.3.6.1 In comparison with other EC countries, the USA and Australia, Figure 2.43 shows that the UK has relatively low consumption of fruit and vegetables (excluding potatoes), pulses, meat and cheese; a relatively high consumption of potatoes and about average consumption of cereals, sugar, fish, eggs, milk, butter, margarine and fats and oils. The consumption of fruit and vegetables in the UK is considerably lower than in countries such as Greece and Italy (370 g/day vs. around 800 g/day). The OECD Food Supply Statistics suggest that the UK has a relatively low proportion of energy from total fat compared to other countries (see Figure C.1 in Appendix C).

Figure 2.43 Consumption estimates based on food supply for EC countries, USA and Australia

Average for 1979-1988

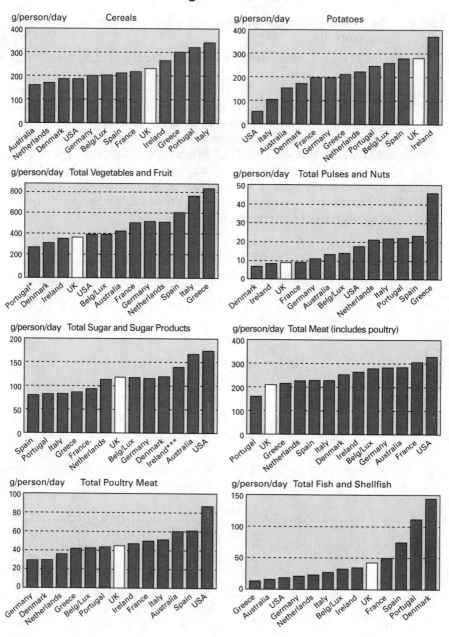

Figure 2.43 *continued*   Consumption estimates based on food supply for EC countries, USA and Australia

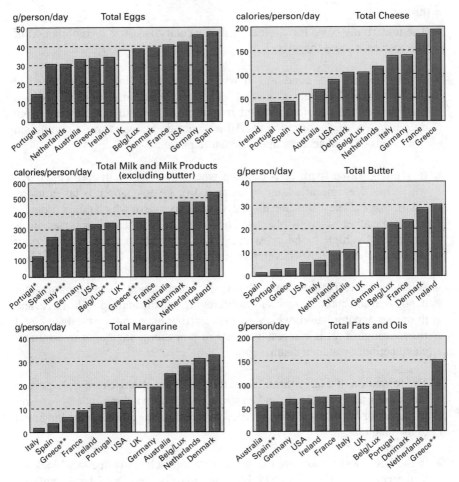

Average for 1979-1988

*average over 9 years
**average over 8 years
***average over 7 years
Belg/Lux = Belgium-Luxembourg Economic Union
NB: Milk and Cheese are given in calories to allow for water content
Source: OECD: Food Consumption Statistics[32]

3. Pathology

Summary

- The underlying basis for clinical cardiovascular disease is a combination of atherosclerosis and thrombosis.

- Atherosclerosis is a condition in which the arterial lining is thickened in places by raised plaques as a result of excessive accumulation of modified lipid and of the proliferation and migration of smooth muscle cells from deeper layers of the artery wall. Atherosclerotic lesions form a continuum from areas of lipid accumulation to mature plaques.

- It is thought that foam cells develop when low density lipoprotein (LDL) which has been modified, eg by oxidation or glycosylation, is taken up by macrophages. These develop into fatty streaks, some of which might progress to become atherosclerotic plaques. The formation of atherosclerotic lesions is promoted by high blood pressure. While fatty streaks are seen in most children, atherosclerosis develops in only a proportion.

- Atherosclerotic plaques grow through a combination of continuing lipid deposition and connective tissue proliferation, and through episodic fibrin and thrombus accumulation, which together narrow the artery and reduce blood flow through it. This can result in new or worsening angina, or intermittent claudication, or sudden death.

- The formation of a large thrombus at the site of an atherosclerotic plaque can block the artery completely and lead to acute myocardial infarction or stroke. In the majority of cases, this is started by a tear or split through the thickness of the plaque.

- In the UK, most strokes are caused by cerebral ischaemia due to a blockage in the cerebral circulation. The blockage may be generated by thrombosis at the site of the ischaemia, or it may arise from the release of thrombus elsewhere in the circulation which then lodges in the heart or neck arteries (embolus). A small proportion of strokes is due to intracerebral or sub-arachnoid haemorrhage.

3.1   Atherosclerosis

3.1.1   Atherosclerosis describes the focal occurrence of raised plaques on the lining of arteries as a result of excessive accumulation of modified lipids, together with proliferation of connective tissue in the arterial wall, which can degenerate at the plaque base.

3.1.2 A lipid rich ("atheromatous") pool forms in the necrotic plaque base; the larger this is in relation to the connective tissue "cap", the greater is the chance of plaque disruption which is the commonest precursor of acute coronary artery thrombosis. Atherosclerotic lesions involve mainly the innermost layer (intima) of the arterial wall, although secondary changes occur in the underlying layer (media). Lesions are focally and not evenly distributed throughout the atherosclerotic tree. The sites of lipid deposition are influenced by characteristics of blood flow and wall stress, and are common at bends and branches.

3.1.3 *The lesions of atherosclerosis* The natural history of atherosclerosis is still not fully known. Fatty streaks are collections of lipid-filled macrophages in the arterial intima and are possible precursors of mature atherosclerotic plaques. They appear early in life and gradually cover more of the arterial surface (see Figure 3.1). There are no significant differences in the extent of fatty streaking between populations with high or low risk of atherosclerosis-related disease[34–38]. Histological assessment of fatty streaks suggests that they are capable of progression to plaque development[39]. The reasons for progression or non-progression are not known.

3.1.4 The more the number of raised plaques, the greater is the risk of atherosclerosis-related clinical events[36,40]. Post-mortem studies show that the number of raised plaques in the coronary arteries increases with the level both of serum low density lipoprotein (LDL) cholesterol concentrations and of cigarette smoking[41].

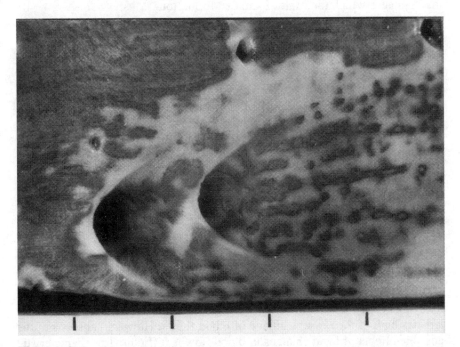

Figure 3.1 *Aorta from a male of 19 years showing extensive fatty streaking. The streak lesions occurring in relation to intercostal arteries are concentrated proximal to the ostia and flow dividers are relatively spared.*

3.1.5 *Lipid modification and accumulation* Like most mammalian tissues the arterial wall contains a considerable amount of lipid which increases with growth and ageing. Atherosclerotic lesions contain far more lipid than normal intima; this lipid accumulates in proportion to the lipid distribution in LDL, suggesting that the latter is of central importance. The entry of LDL into the intima is a necessary, though not sufficient, precondition for lesion formation. Fatty streaks develop when the intra-intimal LDL is taken up by macrophages to form "foam" cells[42].

3.1.6 Macrophages do not take up significant amounts of normal LDL (via the LDL-receptor), but have "scavenger" receptors which recognise the apoprotein of LDL after it has been chemically modified (usually oxidised)[42,43]. Oxidation involves both the apoprotein and the lipid in LDL. It is thought that peroxidation of the lipid in LDL leads to modification of the apoprotein. Polyunsaturated fatty acids are particularly prone to peroxidation (see 4.1.9, 6.5). Once modification of the apoprotein has rendered it recognisable by the scavenger receptor, LDL is taken up avidly by the cells. The effect of this is increasing LDL sequestration in the arterial wall. Oxidation of the lipid in the LDL results also in the formation of a chemoattractant for monocytes, which are not prominent in the normal intima[43,44]. In animal models, antioxidants inhibit lesion development[42,45], but evidence for this in humans, though increasing, is still limited. LDL apoprotein B can also undergo conjugation with glucose to form glycated LDL. The latter appears to be recognised less well by the LDL receptor and is, instead, taken up by macrophages which facilitates foam cell formation[42].

3.1.7 *Intimal connective tissue proliferation* Resting smooth muscle cells are purely contractile, and very few cells actively divide. However, they can be triggered to proliferate when they may show a marked change in function, including production of collagen and other tissue components[46].

3.1.8 *Plaque necrosis* Necrosis at the plaque base, which is associated with increased risk of deep intimal injury and consequent acute thrombosis, is a key event in the natural history of atherosclerosis (see Figure 3.2). Basal necrosis might be accounted for by the presence of macrophages, which can release proteases such as collagenase and elastase, cytokines such as tumour necrosis factor, and oxygen free radicals; but the mechanism of this important phase of the disease and its relationship to factors involved in atherogenesis remains unclear.

3.2   Haemodynamics and atherogenesis

3.2.1   Because of the focal distribution of atherosclerotic plaques, it seems likely that their location and severity is determined to some extent by characteristics both of the vessel wall and of blood flow[47]. However, analysis of the possible effects of local changes in blood flow is difficult. The characteristic distribution pattern, common both to fatty streaks and to mature plaques, suggests that haemodynamic factors may affect mass transport of plasma lipids into the arterial intima.

3.2.2   Three characteristics of flow may affect mass transport: Wall shear rate, which is the velocity gradient between the vessel wall and the centre of the vessel; pressure, which is the stress occurring perpendicular to the surface of the vessel; and shear stress, which is the dragging force acting parallel to the surface of the artery.

3.2.3   Low wall shear rate increases mass transport, as is shown by the relative lack of fatty streaks at the distal portions of branch openings, where the wall shear rate is high. High pressure promotes lesion formation, and those areas of the circulation where pressure is relatively low, such as the pulmonary vasculature, are free from atherosclerosis. Although shear stress is smaller in magnitude than pressure, it may affect not only mass transport but also the function and viability of the endothelial lining, because it is borne directly by the fragile endothelial cells.

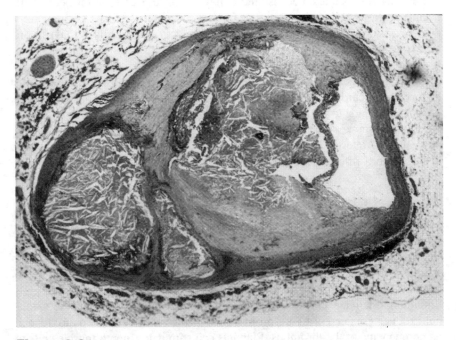

Figure 3.2   *There is an eccentric plaque with one segment of the vessel circumference being free from atherosclerotic changes. The plaque itself shows a complex and massive basal pool of necrotic debris mixed with lipid and the sub-endothelial "cap" is very thin. These features are characteristic of "unstable" plaques which are liable to fissure.*

91

3.3 Thrombosis in relation to atherosclerosis

3.3.1 Coronary heart disease may manifest itself clinically in a number of ways (see section 1.4.1) In stable angina, the coronary arteries typically show one or more segments where the arterial lumen is obstructed by at least 75%. Such lesions are predominantly connective tissue with a small basal atheromatous pool; the connective tissue is often in layers, suggestive of successive episodes of plaque rupture and subsequent healed thrombosis (see 3.3.5). In contrast the other acute, unexpected and life-threatening syndromes are often characterised by acute thrombosis, almost always related to injury of an atheromatous plaque and more irregular lesions.

3.3.2 *Sudden death* Sixty per cent of deaths occurring within six hours of the onset of symptoms are due to CHD[48], although the proportion due to CHD is smaller for deaths occurring within twenty-four hours of the onset of symptoms. CHD is the most common cause of sudden natural death in males and the incidence increases with age. For about half of sudden CHD deaths, no prior symptoms are recorded. Irrespective of the underlying pathology, the common mechanism leading to sudden death related to CHD is abnormal heart rhythms such as ventricular fibrillation.

3.3.3 Pathologically, there are two main groups of patients suffering sudden CHD death. About 70–80% of sudden CHD deaths have been found to have acute coronary artery thrombosis. The heart muscle shows a variable degree of acute ischaemic damage because there may not have been time for necrosis to occur. In cases without evidence of acute thrombosis, there is frequently evidence of healed myocardial infarction; such patients usually have more extensive and severe coronary artery disease.

3.3.4 Clinically the former group are characterised by absence of previous history of myocardial infarction, with a history of preceding chest pain, while the latter group tends to include patients with a history of previous infarction, but without recent chest pain. In these patients with a history of previous infarction, only about a quarter have acute thrombi[49-52]. Sudden death in patients with healed infarcts often results from an abnormal heart rhythm such as ventricular fibrillation[53].

3.3.5 *Effect of thrombosis on the artery wall* Thrombosis may also contribute to plaque growth in atherogenesis, in addition to its role in the acute syndromes[54]. Smooth muscle proliferation is fundamental to atherogenesis and can be accelerated markedly and rapidly by the presence of platelets on an intimal surface[55] (see Figure 3.3). This is most likely following endothelial damage but thrombus-derived emboli also produce intimal thickening[46]. Endothelial damage in the presence of only small numbers of platelets does not produce connective tissue proliferation, which therefore seems to depend on components of the thrombus. Platelets can stimulate smooth muscle cells to proliferate by releasing growth factors, such as platelet derived growth factor and epidermal growth factor.

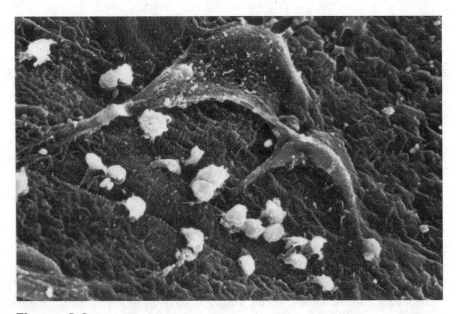

Figure 3.3 *Scanning electron micrograph of a rabbit aorta showing an area of endothelial denudation. Activated platelets are adhering to the exposed sub-endothelial surface.*

3.3.6   The thrombi formed can vary considerably in size. The smaller thrombi, not visible to the naked eye, promote plaque growth. In contrast, the largest are important in the acute syndromes and may also exert a growth promoting effect, leaving survivors with more severe atherosclerotic lesions.

3.3.7   Thrombosis is more likely to occur when there are abnormalities of the vascular wall, of the blood itself and of blood flow. Although the degree of atherosclerosis is related to risk of clinical disease, the characteristics of individual lesions are also important. Thrombosis may occur as a result of a deep tear through the thickness of the plaque into the atheromatous pool, particularly in lesions which are eccentric rather than concentric, and where the basal atheromatous pool is large compared to a thin and easily disrupted connective tissue cap. Such lesions are found in about 75% of acute cases of coronary artery thrombosis. The other 25% occur with superficial plaque injury, where the connective tissue cap is rich in lipid-laden macrophages and, therefore, more fragile.

3.3.8   Blood may be made more liable to thrombosis by abnormalities of platelets and of the clotting and fibrinolytic systems (see section 5.7). Platelets may be more likely to aggregate (as in familial hypercholesterolaemia) and raised plasma levels of some clotting factors (particularly fibrinogen concentration and factor V11c activity) predict risk of the acute syndromes[56]. Cigarette smoking is associated not only with more advanced atherosclerosis, but also with increased plasma fibrinogen concentrations and an increased tendency for platelets to aggregate[57].

3.4 Stroke

3.4.1   Stroke describes focal loss of neurological function of sudden onset, lasting longer than 24 hours, due either to ischaemia or to haemorrhage. The severe, generalized cerebral damage which can occur as a result of hypoxia should not be regarded as stroke.

3.4.2   *Causes of stroke*   The causation of stroke is more complex than CHD, and the importance of various risk factors is not the same for differing causes of stroke. Stroke may be categorised as ischaemic or haemorraghic. Ischaemia causes some 84% of strokes, comprising 53% from in situ thrombosis, and 31% from thrombotic emboli impacting in the cerebral circulation. Emboli may arise from the heart, for instance following a myocardial infarction or other abnormalities, or from atherosclerotic neck arteries. Haemorrhage causes some 16% of strokes; about 10% are intracerebral and 6% are subarachnoid[58].

3.4.3   *Risk factors for stroke*   There are three principal risk factors for stroke.

- The severity of atherosclerosis in the neck and intracranial arteries is of importance for ischaemic stroke. Factors which increase this, in particular cigarette smoking, therefore increase the risk of stroke. Those with ischaemic heart disease have at least a twofold increase in the risk of stroke.

- The presence of high blood pressure is associated with a six-fold increase in the risk of stroke, especially but not solely of haemorrhagic stroke.

- Levels of serum cholesterol less than 5mmol/l are associated with an increased risk of haemorrhagic stroke in people with fairly high blood pressure[59]. The increased risk of haemorrhagic stroke is less than the associated decreased risk of coronary heart disease and thrombotic stroke.

- Diabetes mellitus increases risk principally of ischaemic stroke, possibly through an increase in the extent and severity of atherosclerosis as well as a greater likelihood of high blood pressure due to diabetic renal disease.

- Smoking increases risk of subarachnoid haemorrhage.

3.4.4   *Pathology*   The lesions produced by localised ischaemia, in the brain as in other tissues, are infarcts. These vary greatly in size; some may be only a few millimetres in diameter while others are massive and involve the whole territory of the occluded artery.

3.4.5   It is thought that haemorrhagic stroke occurs as a result of the rupture of aneurysms measuring 1–2mm in diameter found in relation to small intra-cerebral arteries. These aneurysms are present in the brains of 50% of hypertensives, but only 5% of the normotensive population, and 90% of those dying from intra-cerebral haemorrhage. Hypertension appears to be causally related to micro-aneurysms since the number of the latter increases with the duration and severity of the high blood pressure. Rupture of micro-aneurysms causes large intra-cerebral haematomas which tend to track down within the substance of the brain, causing disruption of brain structure and function.

3.4.6   Sub-arachnoid haemorrhage most commonly follows rupture of a congenital aneurysm on one of the major arteries supplying the brain in the layers of tissue surrounding the brain neural tissue. Following a bleed, patients are usually found to be hypertensive, but blood pressure often returns to normal within a few days. There is no clear relationship between sustained hypertension and the risk of rupture, but episodes of high blood pressure may be important.

4.   Biochemistry

Summary

- Fatty acids are molecules made up of a hydrocarbon chain of varying length with a methyl group at one end and a carboxyl group at the other.

- Triglycerides contain three (usually different) fatty acids attached to a glycerol backbone. Mixtures of triglycerides with different fatty acids are the major component of dietary fats.

- Fatty acids are saturated when all carbon atoms in the hydrocarbon chain are attached to 2 hydrogen atoms and are linked by single bonds; monounsaturated if there is one double bond in the hydrocarbon chain; or polyunsaturated if there is more than one double bond in the chain. A double bond is called *cis* if the two hydrogens on each side of the double bond are on the same side of the chain or *trans* if they are on opposite sides of the chain.

- Most of the double bonds in naturally occurring dietary fatty acids are in the *cis* form but *trans* fatty acids are also found in low concentrations in meat and dairy products. Larger amounts of *trans* fatty acids are found in artificially hardened (hydrogenated) fats such as some margarines and shortenings.

- Double bonds are more susceptible to oxidation than single bonds and the more double bonds a fatty acid possesses, the more easily it can be oxidised. Some products of oxidation, oxygen free radicals, can cause cellular and tissue damage if not neutralised by antioxidants.

- Cholesterol is mostly made in the liver (about half to two-thirds) and the rest is provided in the diet. Increasing the amount of cholesterol in the diet decreases the amount synthesized by the liver. Levels of cholesterol in the blood are influenced by the amount and composition of dietary fat and cholesterol, and by constitutional factors including genetic.

- Most cholesterol in the blood is carried in low density lipoprotein (LDL). LDL is taken up from the circulation by binding to specific receptors on cells, especially in the liver. Increasing dietary intakes of saturated fatty acids of chain lengths 12–16 carbon atoms, and of cholesterol, reduces the activity of these receptors and leads to a rise in circulating LDL cholesterol.

- There are two main classes of polyunsaturated fatty acids (n-3 and n-6). Small amounts of linoleic acid (n-6) and alpha linolenic acid (n-3) are essential in the diet as they cannot be synthesized in the body. They can be metabolised to longer chain fatty acids, which are important structural components of cell membranes and can be converted into potent modulators of many metabolic and physiological processes eg prostaglandins.

• Dietary carbohydrates comprise mainly starches and sugars, and non-starch polysaccharides (NSP) which are the main component of dietary fibre. Starches and sugars are digested and absorbed in the small intestine. They are stored in the liver and muscle as glycogen. A number of hormones, particularly insulin, are important in the metabolism of carbohydrates. NSP and some forms of starch are not digested but may be fermented in the large intestine by bacteria. Increasing NSP in the diet leads to increasing stool bulk. Some forms of NSP can help to reduce plasma cholesterol.

4.1   Lipids

4.1.1   Lipids are water-insoluble organic molecules which are classified into complex lipids (eg triglycerides and phospholipids), and simple lipids (e.g. cholesterol).

4.1.2   *Complex lipids*   The fundamental components of complex lipids are fatty acids which comprise a methyl group, a hydrocarbon chain of variable length and a terminal carboxyl group. When each carbon atom of the hydrocarbon chain is attached to two hydrogen atoms, the chain is saturated. Double bonds occur in the chain when single hydrogen atoms on pairs of adjacent carbon atoms are removed. Fatty acids with one double bond are monounsaturated and those with two or more double bonds are polyunsaturated (Figure 4.1). Double bonds influence both the shape of the molecule and the physical and chemical properties of the fatty acid. The chemical terms saturated, monounsaturated and polyunsaturated fatty acids can be abbreviated to saturates, monounsaturates and polyunsaturates, for example, in labelling regulations.

4.1.3   The vast majority of fatty acids in biological systems are bound either to glycerol as triglyceride or to glycerol monophosphate as phospholipid. Triglyceride molecules each contain three fatty acids, usually a mixture of saturated and unsaturated fatty acids. Mixtures of triglycerides with different fatty acids are the major component of dietary fats. Phospholipids contain two fatty acids and are the predominant components of the lipid bilayer of biological membranes. They also stabilize the structure of the lipoproteins which transport lipids in the blood (see below). Membrane phospholipids are a source of the polyunsaturated fatty acids which are precursors of the eicosanoids (e.g. prostaglandins and thromboxanes).

4.1.4   Dietary fatty acids usually contain an even number of carbon atoms (typically 12–24) with up to 4 double bonds. A double bond can adopt two geometrical configurations, denoted 'cis' and 'trans'. In the cis double bond the hydrogen atoms adjacent to the double bond are on the same side of the molecule, while in the trans configuration, they are on opposite sides. Cis double

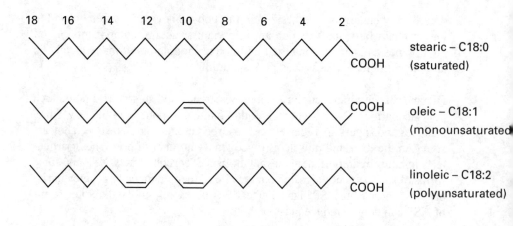

Figure 4.1 Structures for stearic, oleic and linoleic acids *Fatty acids consist of a chain of carbon atoms. In saturates (like stearic acid), all carbons are linked by single bonds. Monounsaturates (like oleic acid) contain one double bond, while polyunsaturates (like linoleic acid) contain two or more. Double bonds influence both the shape of the molecule and the physical and chemical properties of the fatty acid.*

bonds are more common in natural lipids than the trans forms, although trans bonds occur naturally in small amounts in ruminant fats, plant leaf lipids and some seed oils. Double bonds can be located at different positions in the hydrocarbon chain. Conventionally the number of carbon atoms between the methyl terminal of the fatty acid and the first double bond is used to categorise unsaturated fatty acids. Thus where the first double bond is 3 carbons from the methyl terminal, this is termed n-3. During chemical reactions, such as catalytic hydrogenation or oxidation, the double bonds may be shifted along the chain (positional isomerization), or geometrically isomerized (cis-trans), yielding a wider variety of structural isomers than occurs in natural fats and oils (Figure 4.2).

4.1.5   The physical and chemical properties of fatty acids and of the complex lipids derived from them depend on their chain length, degree of saturation, and the nature of any double bonds. The shorter the chain length and the greater the unsaturation, the lower the melting point. Saturated fatty acids and unsaturated fatty acids with trans double bonds are straight and pack closely together. This raises the melting point and tends to make fats containing them more solid at room temperature. Unsaturated fatty acids containing cis double bonds are kinked and less able to pack together. In general, fats with a high proportion of long chain saturated, or trans-unsaturated, fatty acids are solid at room temperature, whereas those with a large number of cis-unsaturated double bonds are liquid oils. Addition of two hydrogens to each double bond in an unsaturated fatty acid converts it into a saturated fatty acid; this is achieved in the industrial process of catalytic hydrogenation in the manufacture of margarine. In practice however, hydrogenation is commonly incomplete, and is then accompanied by the formation of trans double bonds and positional isomerization.

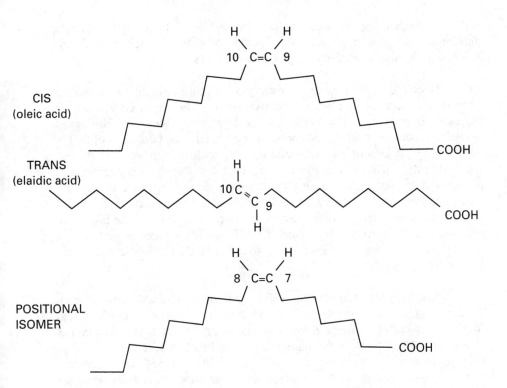

Figure 4.2 Cis, trans and positional isomers of C18:1 fatty acids *Fatty acids with a double bond in the cis configuration are kinked, while those with a trans double bond are straight, like saturated fatty acids. Double bonds may occur not only in different configurations, but also in different positions along the hydrocarbon chain.*

4.1.6   Industrial hydrogenation is not the sole source of dietary trans fatty acids, which have been a small component of the human diet since pre-history. Bacteria in the gastrointestinal tract of ruminants biohydrogenate a large proportion of the unsaturated fatty acids in their diet leading to significant amounts of trans fatty acids in the milk and meat of domesticated animals bred for dairy and beef production[60]. However the main isomers are different from those in artificially hydrogenated fats. Polyunsaturated fatty acids are susceptible to positional isomerization at temperatures of about 180 degrees centigrade reached during deep frying but no significant trans isomerization occurs. At the higher temperatures reached during baking or roasting (220 degrees centigrade), some trans as well as positional isomerization may occur[61,62].

4.1.7   In the United Kingdom, fish oils are still used for the production of margarines and cooking fats although less than previously. Fish oils are more complex than vegetable oils and may contain up to 18% of fatty acids with carbon chains of 20 or more units, with one to six double bonds (compared to less than 1% in vegetable oils)[63]. The variety of positional or geometric isomers which results from their hydrogenation is therefore wider.

4.1.8   Hydrogenation is used not only to process fats for direct human consumption but also for animal food. The trans fatty acids generated find their way into the human food chain via poultry, pork and fish.

4.1.9   Double bonds are more chemically reactive than single bonds and are particularly susceptible to reaction with oxygen to produce a variety of oxidized products that may have important biological properties (see 6.5). Biological oxidation processes result in the continuous production of two kinds of highly reactive oxygen-containing free radicals: the hydroxyl radical (HO•) and superoxide ($0^•_2$). These short-lived intermediates are capable of reacting with polyunsaturated fatty acids, leading to a chain reaction which is greatly accelerated by the presence of metal ions such as iron and copper. If the fatty acid happens to be an integral component of a lipoprotein like LDL, the biological properties of the particle may change[42,64]. These events together may trigger lipoprotein oxidation, leading ultimately to the generation of cholesterol-laden foam cells (see 3.1, 6.5).

4.1.10 *Simple lipids*   Cholesterol is the most abundant simple lipid in man. All animal cells need cholesterol, derived both from endogenous synthesis and from the diet, both for structural and for metabolic purposes. In cell membranes it helps to maintain appropriate fluidity for normal function of membrane-linked enzyme systems and transport proteins. In specialised tissues like the adrenal glands, gonads and liver, it is a precursor of adrenocortical hormones, sex steroids and bile acids respectively.

4.1.11 *Lipid metabolism*   The UK diet provides about 200-300 times more complex lipid (triglycerides) than simple lipid (cholesterol), an average of about 70–100 g of triglyceride and about 250–400 mg of cholesterol daily[4] (see 2.3). Endogenous synthesis generates some 450 mg (12 mmol) of cholesterol daily. Dietary cholesterol absorption varies markedly between individuals[65]. Triglyceride is almost completely absorbed. Lipids are carried in the blood in specialised proteins called lipoproteins. In the gut wall, dietary lipids are incorporated into large triglyceride-rich lipoproteins (chylomicrons) which are secreted into the circulation. There the triglyceride is hydrolysed by lipoprotein lipase on capillary endothelium and its constituent fatty acids and glycerol released for storage or energy needs (Figure 4.3). Chylomicron remnants containing the dietary derived cholesterol are rapidly assimilated by the liver. A by product of this process is high density lipoprotein (HDL) which is important in transporting cholesterol from the periphery to the liver (see 4.1.13). Increasing the dietary cholesterol absorbed and delivered to the liver decreases its endogenous synthesis. Dietary derived cholesterol in excess of hepatic capacity to assimilate chylomicron remnants is secreted into the bile as well as the plasma, so that *plasma* cholesterol is only partly influenced by *dietary* cholesterol intake.

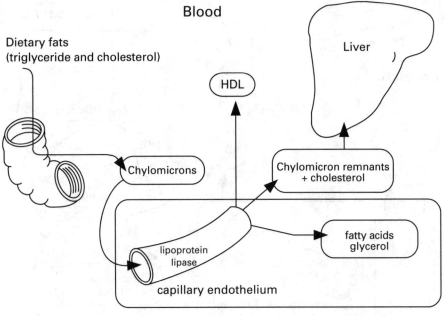

Blood

Dietary fats
(triglyceride and cholesterol)

HDL

Liver

Chylomicrons

Chylomicron remnants
+ cholesterol

fatty acids
glycerol

lipoprotein
lipase

capillary endothelium

adipose tissue / skeletal muscle

Figure 4.3 Exogenous lipid metabolism *Following absorption, dietary fat is transported in the circulation in large triglyceride-rich particles (chylomicrons). There, lipolysis reduces the particle's triglyceride core and makes redundant part of its surface coat which is shed as high density lipoprotein (HDL). The chylomicron remnants produced in the process containing dietary derived cholesterol are rapidly assimilated by the liver. Arrows indicate transit through the vascular compartment.*

4.1.12 Except after a meal, the liver secretes triglyceride-rich particles (Very Low Density Lipoproteins; VLDL) to supply the tissues (Figure 4.4). Hydrolysis in the tissues releases fatty acids from triglycerides and produces a cholesterol-rich remnant (Low Density Lipoprotein; LDL) via an intermediate species, intermediate density lipoprotein (IDL). In contrast to the rapid clearance from the circulation of chylomicron remnants, LDL is cleared only relatively slowly by specific LDL receptors. The activity of these receptors on all cells is regulated by the intracellular need for cholesterol, and is a key determinant of the plasma concentration of LDL-cholesterol[66]. The liver is particularly rich in LDL receptors. Increasing dietary intake of saturated fatty acids of chain lengths 12–16 appears to down-regulate the activity of these receptors (Figure 4.5).

4.1.13 Cholesterol in excess of cellular need is transported to the liver in a process called reverse cholesterol transport. High density lipoprotein (HDL) appears to act as a primary acceptor of tissue cholesterol and transfers it on to IDL which ultimately delivers it to the liver either via LDL receptors or directly. Imbalance in the system, as yet inadequately defined, may lead to the uptake of LDL cholesterol by a non-saturable "scavenger" receptor on macrophages in the vascular wall. This process may require prior modification of the LDL, eg by oxidation, which might be a key initiating stage in the development of atherosclerosis[42] (see 3.1, 6.5).

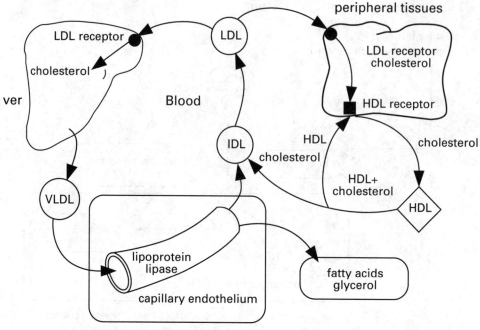

Figure 4.4 Endogenous lipid metabolism and reverse cholesterol transport *Except after a meal, very low density lipoprotein (VLDL) are the major triglyceride transporters. They too are subject to tissue lipolysis which degrades them to low density lipoproteins (LDL) via an intermediate species (IDL). The LDL is removed by receptors on liver and peripheral tissues. When these are saturated, an alternative, scavenger pathway becomes dominant. Arrows indicate transit through the vascular compartment. High density lipoproteins (HDL) retrieve cholesterol from peripheral tissue and promote its transfer (via LDL) to the liver.*

4.1.14   *n-6 and n-3 polyunsaturated fatty acids*   The essential fatty acids are linoleic acid (C18:2 n-6) and alpha linolenic acid (C18:3 n-3). These are elongated and desaturated by a series of enzymes and converted to their longer chain derivatives, arachidonic acid (C20:4 n-6), and eicosapentaenoic (C20:5 n-3) (EPA) and docosahexaenoic (C22:6 n-3) (DHA) respectively. Oils from corn, safflower, sunflower and soyabean are rich sources of linoleic acid. Soyabean and rapeseed oils are good sources of alpha linolenic acid, and fish, particularly oily fish, good sources of EPA and DHA.

4.1.15   When incorporated in cell membrane phospholipids, these polyunsaturated fatty acids are the source of C20 unsaturated fatty acids for the production of a group of highly active metabolic products called eicosanoids, which include the prostanoids (prostaglandins and thromboxanes). In platelets, binding of certain agonists such as collagen to surface receptors stimulates the release of arachidonic acid, a precursor of thromboxane A_2[67], which is a potent platelet activating agent and a potent vasoconstrictor[68] (see 6.3).

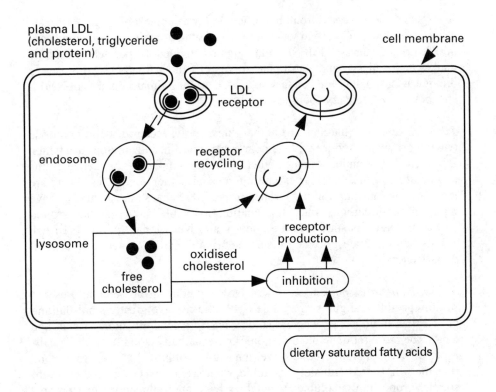

Figure 4.5 Plasma cholesterol levels and the LDL receptor *The Low Density Lipoprotein (LDL) receptor is central to the regulation of plasma cholesterol levels. When intracellular cholesterol levels are low, the number of receptors on the cell membrane rises, and more LDL is taken up. Delivery of the lipoprotein (triglycerides + cholesterol + binding apoprotein) to lysosomes results in the release of free cholesterol (or an oxidised derivative) which then suppresses further receptor production and so modulates LDL uptake by the cell. Dietary saturated fatty acids may also down-regulate receptor production, thereby increasing plasma LDL levels by inhibiting its catabolism.*

4.2 Carbohydrates

4.2.1 Carbohydrates provide a major part of the food energy in most human diets, ranging from around 45 per cent in industrialised countries to 85 per cent in developing countries. Dietary carbohydrates comprise mainly starches and sugars, but also include non-starch polysaccharides (NSP), the main component of dietary fibre. Starches and sugars are digested in the small intestine and made available as a source of energy to the tissues. NSP and some starches (resistant starch) are not utilised in this way, but can undergo fermentation in the large intestine to form short-chain fatty acids which can be utilised as a source of energy.

4.2.2 *Sugars* Sugars are soluble oligosaccharides, principally monosaccharides and disaccharides, of which the most abundant in nature is the monosaccharide glucose. Other common monosaccharides are fructose and galactose, and common disaccharides are sucrose, maltose and lactose. Dietary sugars have been classified into intrinsic and extrinsic[69]. Intrinsic sugars are those naturally present and embodied in the cellular structure of food, and extrinsic sugars those separated from this structure, for example table sugar. Extrinsic sugars in milk were classified separately and all others of this type are called non-milk extrinsic sugars (NMES). Total sugars provided 18 per cent of energy intakes in the Dietary and Nutritional Survey of British Adults[4]. NMES usually provide at least half of total dietary sugars[2]. Current estimated intakes of NMES are about 13% of dietary energy (see 2.3).

4.2.3   *Starches*   Starches are alpha-glucan polysaccharides and comprise two major types: amylose with a linear configuration, and amylopectin which is branched. The major sources of dietary starches in the UK are cereal grains and potatoes, and to a lesser extent legumes and other vegetables. There are few data on consumption of starches in the UK because most surveys have reported total carbohydrate. Information available suggests that around half of the latter is starch. In the Dietary and Nutritional Survey of British Adults carbohydrate provided 42 per cent, and starch 24 per cent, of total dietary energy[4].

4.2.4   *Non-starch polysaccharides*   NSP includes insoluble celluloses and soluble pectins and gums. Insoluble NSP tend to have greater stool-bulking effects than soluble NSP, whereas soluble NSP are generally more viscous and tend to be more fermentable by colonic bacteria than insoluble NSP. Cereals, especially whole grain products, are rich sources of NSP. In wheat, maize and rice, the NSP is predominately insoluble, whereas in oats, rye and barley a substantial proportion is soluble. Vegetables have approximately equal proportions of soluble and insoluble NSP. Average intakes of NSP in the UK are 12g/day[31], about half provided by cereals and half by vegetables[4].

4.2.5   *Metabolism of starches and sugars*   After digestion dietary carbohydrate is absorbed and delivered as glucose or fructose to the liver where fructose is rapidly converted either to glucose or to lactate. At least half the glucose passes through the liver unchanged and is taken up by peripheral tissues, primarily muscle, where it is deposited as glycogen. Of the rest, some is deposited as liver glycogen, and some is converted to fatty acids via glycolysis and secreted as VLDL-triglyceride (see 4.1.12). In the fasting state glycogen is broken down in the liver (glycogenolysis) and released as glucose for use by the brain and other tissues. Glucose is also formed *de novo* from lactate, amino acids and glycerol in the liver (gluconeogenesis).

4.2.6   *Insulin*   All these processes are under hormonal control. In the fasting state insulin levels are low, and the actions of the catabolic hormones (glucagon, cortisol and catecholamines) predominate, promoting glycogenolysis and gluconeogenesis in liver; increased adipose tissue lipolysis with release of free fatty acids and ultimately ketone bodies into the circulation; and net negative protein balance. When insulin levels rise, such as after a meal, hepatic glucose output is suppressed and carbohydrate is stored as glycogen. Excess glucose is converted into fatty acids and triglycerides in the liver and transported to adipose tissue in VLDL (see 4.1.12). Lipoprotein lipase cleaves VLDL to release fatty acids which then enter adipocytes. In smooth muscle and arterial walls insulin can act as a growth promoting factor increasing, for example, smooth muscle cell proliferation[70]. It also increases smooth muscle tone and enhances sodium reabsorption by the kidney.

4.2.7   The primary regulator of insulin secretion is the level of plasma glucose. If the tissues including the liver are resistant to the action of insulin then hepatic glucose output is not suppressed, peripheral glucose disposal is poor, and plasma glucose levels rise, further stimulating insulin secretion. The resulting hyper-insulinaemia occurs in a variety of insulin resistant states which are associated with increased risk of cardiovascular disease, most strikingly in non-insulin dependent diabetes mellitus (See 5.6).

4.2.8   *NSP and metabolism*   The laxative effect of NSP has been well documented. In healthy people there is a simple linear relation between NSP intake and stool weight over a range of 4-32 g/d^2. Cell wall polysaccharides may also reduce the utilization of energy from foods. NSP in intact foods contributes to satiety and reduces the post-prandial fluctuations of plasma glucose and insulin levels[2,71]. In addition, some soluble forms of NSP such as guar and pectin lower plasma cholesterol through mechanisms not known[2]. The amount of NSP required for a biologically significant effect depends on its nature, and therefore on its food source (see 6.4).

5. Major factors which affect risk of cardiovascular disease

Summary

- Numerous epidemiological and clinical studies have demonstrated a strong, continuous and positive relationship between plasma total cholesterol and risk of CHD. The relationship resides mainly in the low density lipoprotein (LDL) fraction, which carries most of the cholesterol in the blood.

- Lowering raised plasma cholesterol by diet or drugs lowers risk of CHD. Although direct evidence for this is mainly from trials in middle aged men, a variety of observational data are consistent, and indicate that men and women, young and older, would benefit from having lower plasma cholesterol levels.

- A 1 per cent lower plasma total cholesterol translates into a 2 to 3 per cent lower risk of CHD. A reduction in plasma cholesterol can slow down the rate of progression and may induce regression of coronary atherosclerosis. Increasing levels of plasma high density lipoprotein (HDL) cholesterol is associated with decreased risk of death from CHD in Western populations.

- A J-shaped relationship between plasma total cholesterol and non cardio-vascular and total mortality is seen in many prospective and intervention studies, ie. at the lowest levels of blood cholesterol, mortality rates are higher than at slightly higher levels. However there is no consistent indication of increased mortality rates in populations with low average blood cholesterol. Increased mortality at low cholesterol levels could be explained by pre-existing disease at the time of initial cholesterol measurement, or to confounding by lifestyle factors. In trials of cholesterol lowering, only drug treatment was associated with increased non-cardiovascular mortality. Current evidence suggests that the beneficial effects in the population which would be expected from the changes recommended in this report, and which would lower the average plasma cholesterol, outweigh any potential adverse effect in the minority of the population with the lowest plasma cholesterol levels.

- Risk of stroke and CHD increases with the level of blood pressure, and sustained reduction of raised levels lowers the incidence of both conditions. Higher levels of blood pressure within the conventional "normal" range are important because they are common, and contribute the majority of deaths and non-fatal cardiovascular events attributable to raised blood pressure.

- Obesity is one of the commonest and most easily recognised causes of ill health. Obesity increases risk of CHD, respiratory disease, diabetes, gall bladder disease, and some cancers. The distribution of fat about the body also influences risk: excessive abdominal fat is associated with greater risk of CHD than excessive fatness of the hips and thighs. Weight loss has beneficial effects on blood pressure, blood lipids, and insulin resistance. However, treatment of obesity is often difficult, and may itself be associated with adverse effects; prevention is therefore of special importance.

- Diabetes mellitus is associated with a large excess risk of cardiovascular disease. Lesser degrees of disordered carbohydrate metabolism, thought to be linked to insulin resistance, are associated with the presence of obesity, hypertension and dyslipidaemia, and also increased risk of cardiovascular disease.

- Abnormalities of haemostasis, e.g. plasma fibrinogen and factor VII, and of thrombosis, e.g. platelet function, can increase risk of CHD events.

- Cigarette smoking powerfully increases incidence of CHD, stroke and peripheral vascular disease in both sexes. The more cigarettes smoked, the higher is the risk. Middle aged smokers have about double the risk of a major coronary event as non-smokers. If risk is elevated because of other risk factors, smoking increases the risk further. In particular, smoking substantially increases the very small risk in young women using oral contraceptives. The mechanisms by which smoking promotes cardiovascular disease are uncertain. Smokers tend to have unfavourable blood lipid patterns and higher fibrinogen levels. Smoking also increases the requirement for antioxidant nutrients, while their intake by smokers tends to be low.

- Physical inactivity is linked to an increased risk of CHD, but only a minority of adults currently take sufficient exercise to benefit their health. Simple forms of exercise like walking, cycling and swimming are likely to be effective in decreasing risk of CHD. Physical exercise can help to maintain desirable body weight, and has beneficial effects on blood pressure, insulin sensitivity and possibly blood coagulation mechanisms. Exercise need not be of high intensity to confer benefit.

5.1   **Introduction**   This section addresses a number of factors which are associated with the risk of cardiovascular disease. There are many known associations with cardiovascular risk (see 1.5.15–18), ranging from psychosocial to biological. These, and in particular, the important contribution which genetic factors make to individual CHD risk, and so to the variation of risk within a population, are not considered here except insofar as dietary or nutritional factors impinge on them. In spite of their potential relevance to individual risk, there is no evidence that genetic factors are responsible for the differences in CHD risk between populations. Furthermore, genetic predisposition is not, currently, either reliably identifiable or susceptible to modification. In addition, since the cumulated effect of known risk factors does not appear to explain all the variance in cardiovascular disease occurrence, other unknown factors may also operate. The factors identified here are those where dietary or nutritional factors may be relevant. It is not intended to be a comprehensive list of all known factors affecting cardiovascular risk.

5.2   Plasma lipids

5.2.1   Longitudinal studies of individuals from several countries demonstrate a strong, positive and curvilinear relation between plasma cholesterol concentration and the incidence of CHD; those with higher mean cholesterol concentrations experience higher CHD mortality[71-76]. A similar relation can be demonstrated between populations and in migrants; migrants usually acquire similar plasma cholesterol levels to the native population and a similar CHD risk[77,78]. This relation between plasma cholesterol and CHD resides mainly within the low density lipoprotein (LDL) fraction, which carries most of plasma total cholesterol. The cholesterol:CHD relationship is present throughout the range of plasma cholesterol observed in diverse populations. In parts of China mean cholesterol is about 3.3 mmol/L, in Japan mean cholesterol is about 4.9 mmol/d[79,80], but even at these lower levels, individuals with lower plasma cholesterol levels have lower CHD risk than those with higher cholesterol levels, as in the UK; however these low cholesterol countries have a much lower overall incidence of CHD. Patients with familial hypercholesterolaemia are at the top of the cholesterol distribution. Many heterozygous individuals suffer a myocardial infarction before 50 years of age. In homozygotes this may occur during adolescence[81,82]. The strength of the association between plasma cholesterol and future coronary risk is greater in younger people. An analysis of the 10 largest prospective studies found that a 10% reduction in serum cholesterol was associated with a 54% reduction in the incidence of CHD at 40 years and a 19% reduction at 80 years[12]. In older people the relative risk may be less in part because of lifestyle changes and premature CHD death among the most susceptible.

5.2.2   Epidemiological studies generally employ only a single baseline estimate of plasma cholesterol concentration. The effect of within-person variation in plasma cholesterol on the estimate of the relation between cholesterol-lowering and reduction in CHD introduces an error which results in an underestimation of risk (regression dilution bias)[83]. The correlation within individuals between repeated plasma cholesterol measures some time apart is about 0.7. The estimated true reduction in coronary risk associated with a 1% reduction in plasma cholesterol concentration, after adjustment for errors in variables, approaches 3%, compared to the 2% observed in the unadjusted data from epidemiological studies[13,83].

5.2.3   The effectiveness of lowering plasma cholesterol in reducing CHD risk has been examined in a number of intervention trials, some of which have aimed simply to reduce plasma cholesterol, while others have been of multifactorial design. Plasma cholesterol has been lowered either by diet alone, or by drugs, or by a combination of these approaches. In one overview analysis of 22 trials which intervened on plasma cholesterol alone either by dietary or drug therapy, for primary or secondary prevention, treatment produced an overall reduction of 23% in risk of an acute coronary event (95% confidence interval – 18% to 28%)[84]. The effect of therapy was related directly to the degree and duration of plasma cholesterol lowering. In 14 trials of under 4 years duration, a 10% reduction in plasma cholesterol led to a 10% reduction in risk, compared with a 20% reduction in the 8 trials of more prolonged intervention[84]. An analysis of 28 trials by Law et al showed that the full effect of the reduction in risk is achieved by 5 years, when the achieved reduction is similar to that observed in prospective studies[12,13]. In another overview which included plasma cholesterol lowering trials that intervened against additional risk factors such as blood pressure and smoking[85], a similar result was obtained, a 1% reduction in plasma cholesterol being associated with about a 2.5% reduction in risk of an acute coronary event (95% confidence interval, 1.1% to 3.9%). In both analyses, reduction in CHD incidence by plasma cholesterol lowering did not appear to differ between primary and secondary prevention trials; also, single and multifactorial trials appeared to be similarly effective in this respect[85].

5.2.4   These randomised trials provide direct information mostly in middle aged men with baseline plasma cholesterol concentrations of 6.4 mmol/L (247 mg/dl) or more, treated for about 1 to 7 years. There are no directly comparable data with which to assess the effects of longer intervention in younger patients, or in those with lower levels of plasma cholesterol. Where they overlap in duration of follow-up, however, the observational and interventional studies are consistent. It therefore seems likely that the results from these studies are broadly generalisable to other population groups.

5.2.5   *Lipoprotein cholesterol*   Most evidence relating plasma cholesterol to CHD risk concerns levels of total plasma cholesterol. However plasma cholesterol comprises a number of subfractions (see 4.1). There is now good evidence that the different subfractions carry different implications for CHD risk. The major portion of total cholesterol is carried on low density lipoprotein (LDL cholesterol). Most of the remainder is carried on high density lipoprotein (HDL cholesterol). There is less evidence linking LDL and HDL cholesterol than total cholesterol to cardiovascular risk as early studies did not measure them. The differences in total cholesterol between populations are principally due to differences in LDL cholesterol[86].

5.2.5.1   *LDL cholesterol*   There is substantial evidence that the association between total cholesterol and CHD risk is mediated largely through LDL cholesterol. An association between LDL cholesterol and CHD risk in different populations has been demonstrated in a number of studies. In addition, several prospective studies have demonstrated a positive association between baseline LDL cholesterol and subsequent CHD risk[86]. Reduction of LDL cholesterol is associated with reduced CHD risk (see 5.2.6).

5.2.5.2   *HDL cholesterol*   HDL cholesterol varies less than LDL cholesterol between populations and the average level of HDL cholesterol within a population is not consistently associated with CHD risk. In contrast, HDL cholesterol in individuals within Western populations is inversely associated with CHD risk, although this has not been a universal finding[86,87]. The mechanism of the inverse association between HDL cholesterol and CHD risk is not clear and the influence of HDL cholesterol on CHD risk is only apparent where mean LDL cholesterol levels are high. The ratio of HDL to either total or LDL cholesterol is sometimes used as a combined marker of CHD risk, although its clinical value is limited by difficulty in interpretation.

5.2.6   Early attempts to demonstrate retardation or regression of coronary atherosclerosis, as assessed by angiography, following plasma cholesterol lowering by dietary, drug[89] or surgical intervention[89] were flawed because of lack of statistical power, crudeness of angiographic techniques, and absence of suitable controls. In three more recent trials of lipid lowering therapy in patients with angiographically demonstrated coronary atherosclerosis and hyperlipidaemia, all double-blind, placebo-controlled and with randomised allocation to treatment or control group, treatment for between 2 and 5 years significantly retarded the rate of coronary stenosis[90–92]. In a further study, men advised to follow a lipid-lowering diet and those on diet and cholestyramine showed a lower incidence of progression and a higher incidence of luminal widening compared to controls after 3 years as assessed by coronary angiography[93]. In another study, myocardial infarction survivors with resistant hypercholesterolaemia were randomised either to a low-fat diet alone or to have in addition a partial ileal bypass. Coronary stenosis on angiography, as well as the incidence both of non-fatal and fatal acute coronary events, were significantly reduced in the surgical group[95] over an average follow-up of almost 10 years. In all five trials retardation of stenosis was accompanied by reductions in plasma LDL cholesterol concentrations, and a small but significant increase in HDL cholesterol[90–94].

5.2.7   *Plasma cholesterol and total and non-cardiovascular mortality*
5.2.7.1 A J-shaped association between plasma cholesterol and total mortality has been observed in a number of prospective studies and meta-analyses of studies and has raised concern that low plasma cholesterol levels might be associated with increased rates of mortality from stroke, cancer and other non-cardiovascular causes such as suicide, chronic bronchitis and chronic liver and bowel diseases[95]. It was suggested that the original reported association between low plasma cholesterol and colon cancer mortality[96] might be a consequence of pre-existing but undiagnosed cancer at the time of plasma cholesterol measurement[97]. This possibility was explored in a number of studies in middle aged men by excluding deaths occurring within the first few years after cholesterol measurement, the assumption being that pre-existing cancers would be fatal within a few years. Excluding early deaths attenuated or abolished the relationship in some but not all studies. These studies all linked plasma cholesterol levels in middle age with subsequent mortality. However in a study which related plasma cholesterol in young men to later cardiovascular and other mortality, low initial plasma cholesterol concentrations were not associated with increased mortality[98].

5.2.7.2 The US National Heart, Lung and Blood Institute (NHLBI) has published a statistical overview of data from the majority of large prospective studies in this area[95]. This found a J-shaped relationship between total cholesterol and total mortality in men, but essentially no relationship in women after excluding deaths in the first 5 years. There was an increased risk of death due to a variety of causes in men with plasma cholesterol levels less than 4.1 mmol/L, ie in the bottom 6% of the distribution. The strength, gradation and persistence of the individual relationships varied. An analysis by Law et al found that excess mortality associated with levels of serum cholesterol less than 5mmol/L was not seen in studies of employed men but was restricted to studies of community cohorts who are likely to include larger numbers with pre-existing illness[59]. Haemorrhagic stroke was the only cause of death attributable to low serum cholesterol concentration.

5.2.7.3 A number of explanations could account for the observed associations[99]. Pre-existing disease probably accounts for a proportion of the increased deaths and may not be completely allowed for by excluding deaths in the first 5 years. Cancers of the haemopoietic systems, especially leukaemia, lead to low plasma cholesterol levels, and successful treatment results in a rise in plasma cholesterol levels[100,101]. Chronic illness could cause reductions in plasma cholesterol levels and be associated with increased mortality risk[102]. For diseases such as respiratory illness or chronic hepatitis and for some cancers[103], there is a long clinical course between the development of symptoms and death. Exclusion of early deaths does not, therefore, exclude the possibility that pre-existing disease is a common factor leading both to low plasma cholesterol levels and to increased mortality rates. The lack of effect in studies in employed men is further evidence that pre-existing disease could account for much of the observed associations[59].

5.2.7.4 The persistence of some of the observed relationships, however, raises the possibility that pre-existing disease cannot account for all the increased mortality. Another possible explanation is confounding by a third factor, related both to low plasma cholesterol and to increased mortality. In some cohorts, the causes of death which are elevated among subjects with low plasma cholesterol levels tend to be those which are related to low socio-economic status. In the Whitehall study, where men in lower civil service employment grades had lower plasma cholesterol levels and higher rates of mortality from respiratory and digestive disease, adjusting for employment grade, as an index of socio-economic status led to attenuation of the association between low plasma cholesterol level and elevated mortality. Confounding by socio-economic status is likely to occur in other cohorts[104].

5.2.7.5 A third possible explanation of the observed associations is that there is a direct causal relationship between low plasma cholesterol and increased mortality. Cholesterol is known to have general, fundamental and highly specific roles in the body; for example, it affects the fluidity of cell membranes, membrane permeability, signal transmission, and acts as a precursor for five classes of steroid hormones. Low levels of plasma cholesterol could conceivably have widespread effects in the body. However, there is no evidence that the levels of cholesterol associated with increased mortality cause cellular dysfunction and the apparent safety, for instance in the Chinese, of levels considered low in European populations also argues against this. Furthermore, the absolute level of plasma cholesterol at which the increased risk of non-cardiovascular death is seen varies across populations. In Scotland it was only seen below 5.0 mmol/L[105] and in China, only below 3.5 mmol/L[20]. The causes of death also vary. In China, low plasma cholesterol is associated with increased primary liver cancer – a cause of death that was not seen in British studies. These findings suggest that excess risk among the minority of people at the low end of any cholesterol distribution may result from factors other than the level of cholesterol itself.

5.2.7.6 An increase in mortality due to non-cardiovascular, non-cancer deaths, particularly accidents, violence and suicide, has also been observed in the intervention groups of cholesterol-lowering intervention trials and in meta-analyses of these trials[102,106–108]. *Falling* plasma cholesterol levels might have different biological effects from *consistently* low levels, or the means of lowering plasma cholesterol used in intervention studies could itself lead to increased mortality risk. An analysis of cholesterol-lowering trials by diet and drugs found an increase in non-cardiovascular deaths restricted to the drug trials only[102] and an analysis according to the level of risk of CHD in the control population found that cholesterol-lowering resulted in a significant reduction in total mortality only in populations at an initially high risk of CHD. The extent of the reduction in cholesterol was not related to deaths from non-coronary causes suggesting that cholesterol reduction *per se* is unlikely to cause increased non-cardiovascular mortality[108]. A further analysis by Law *et al*[59], which also found significant excess mortality in the intervention groups of drug trials, argues that the excess deaths occurred predominantly among men who did not take the treatment or who had psychiatric illness already and that apart from 9 deaths attributable to known adverse effect of specific treatments, there was no evidence of an increased mortality from any cause arising specifically from reduction in cholesterol concentration *per se*. Nevertheless, the side effects of each cholesterol lowering drug should be monitored individually.

5.2.8 *Conclusions* Evidence for the role of plasma cholesterol as a determinant of CHD risk is derived from a variety of sources. Both the epidemiological evidence from populations and experimental studies in individuals favour a direct contributory role for plasma cholesterol, and in particular, LDL cholesterol, in the causation of CHD. Some, but not all, prospective studies have shown an association between low plasma total cholesterol at initial examination and increased total and non-cardiovascular mortality at follow up, and trials of cholesterol-lowering drugs have also found increased mortality in the intervention groups. The reasons for these two observations may be different. In prospective studies at least some of the increased mortality associated with low cholesterol can be attributed to pre-existing disease or confounding. Increased non-cardiovascular mortality is not found in populations with low average concentrations of plasma cholesterol. There is no evidence that lifelong low plasma cholesterol, rather than more short term reduction of plasma cholesterol in middle age, is associated with adverse effects. While a cautious approach to the clinical treatment of certain individuals already at increased risk seems justified, the dietary patterns recommended in this Report can safely be adopted with benefit for the whole population.

5.2.9 *Lipoprotein (a)* Lipoprotein(a) or Lp(a) is a variant of LDL; it closely resembles LDL but it contains an additional protein known as apoprotein(a) or apo(a). Apo(a) is very similar in structure to plasminogen, the precursor of plasmin, which converts insoluble fibrin to soluble fibrin degradation products (see 5.7). Plasma Lp(a) concentrations are largely under genetic control and vary widely in the population. High plasma Lp(a) levels have been associated in retrospective epidemiological studies with an increased incidence of athero-sclerotic cardiovascular disease, particularly in people under 60 years[109–111] but not in prospective studies[112,113]. The unique structural features of Lp(a) with similarities both to LDL and to plasminogen may be important. Like LDL it can be chemically modified and taken up by the scavenger-receptor pathway on macrophages[114]. It can also compete with tissue plasminogen activator, which converts plasminogen to plasmin (see 5.7)[115] and therefore might interfere with the fibrinolytic process. Recent studies have suggested that trans fatty acids might influence Lp(a) levels (see 6.2.6).

5.3   Blood pressure

5.3.1 *Systolic and diastolic blood pressure* are directly related to the risk of coronary heart disease and stroke[116]. An overview analysis of 9 prospective studies, which together followed about 420,000 adults (96% men) for an average of 10 years, showed the relation between CHD and stroke incidence and diastolic blood pressure to be linear, positive and continuous across the range of pressures studied[117]. When adjustments were made for the unreliability of the single baseline estimate of blood pressure as a guide to an individual's usual pressure and for the effects of blood cholesterol, smoking and age, a 7.5 mmHg difference in diastolic pressure within the range 70–110 mmHg was accompanied by a 29% difference in CHD risk, and a 46% difference in risk of stroke, irrespective of sex, age group or ethnicity[117]. The association almost certainly arises through enhancement of several components of cardiovascular pathology by raised blood pressure (see Chapter 3)[118].

5.3.2 *Blood pressure and stroke* Reducing blood pressure leads to reduced risk of stroke. The overview of nine prospective trials[117] found that a difference of 5mmHg in diastolic blood pressure was associated with at least 34% less stroke. In an overview of 14 randomised trials of anti-hypertensive drugs, in which the mean reduction in diastolic blood pressure was 5–6mmHg over 5 years, stroke was reduced by 42%. This suggests that virtually all the epidemiologically expected stroke reduction appears rapidly[119].

5.3.3   Sustained reduction of raised blood pressures by hypotensive agents reduces the incidence of CHD. In an examination of the overall results of 14 ran-domised trials of antihypertensive drug therapy, involving 37,000 individuals (mostly with baseline diastolic blood pressures < 110 mm Hg) who were followed for 5 years on average, a 5–6 mm Hg reduction in diastolic pressure was associated with a 14% reduction in acute coronary events. This effect was statistically significant and appeared to apply similarly to mild, mild-to-moderate, and more severe grades of hypertension[119]. Most of this benefit was observed within 1–2 years of starting treatment.

5.3.4   For the individual patient, the importance of hypertension is directly related to the degree of elevation of the blood pressure. For the community, the more important burden of hypertension-related morbidity comes from higher levels of blood pressure within the conventionally accepted normal range than from more severe grades, because they are much more common and account for the majority of deaths and non-fatal clinical events attributable to raised blood pressure (see 1.5.10).

5.4   Obesity

5.4.1   Obesity is one of the commonest and most easily recognised causes of ill-health in the UK. In addition to its role in cardiovascular disease it contributes to morbidity and mortality from respiratory disease, diabetes, gall bladder disease and some cancers. In adults, a useful surrogate for direct measurement of body fatness is the body mass index (BMI), which is weight (kg) divided by height (m)^2. Categories of BMI suggested for the UK are: under 20: underweight; 20-25: normal (desirable) range; 25–30: overweight; above 30: obese. The BMI takes no account of body fat distribution. In England between 1980 and 1991, the proportion of adults with a BMI between 25–30 increased from 35 to 40 per cent of men and from 24 to 26 per cent of women. The proportion of men with a BMI over 30 increased from 6 to 13 per cent, and of women from 8 to 15 per cent. The relationship between diet and obesity is discussed in Section 6.8.

5.4.2   The incidence of CHD is high in obese men and women, particularly in those under 50 years of age. There is a graded increase in the risk of cardiovascular and total mortality with increasing BMI above about 25[120]. The association is increasingly apparent when incidence is measured over a decade or more rather than over shorter periods[121–124]. In addition to fatness per se, the distribution of fat about the body also influences risk of CHD. Men and women with excessive abdominal fat (central obesity) are at greater risk than those of similar fat mass in which the distribution is more peripheral (about the hips and thighs)[125–127]. Even when of lesser degree, overweight is associated with a cluster of characteristics which in themselves raise the risk of CHD (see 5.6.4).

5.4.3   Change in degree of adiposity during younger adult life has been shown to be related to changes in related risk factors[128–129]. Weight loss has beneficial effects on blood pressure, plasma lipids and insulin resistance[129,130]. However, repeated cycles of weight loss and weight gain may incur an additional risk to health[131–133]. Further research is needed in this area.

5.4.4   The fundamental metabolic defect following from central obesity may be reduced sensitivity to insulin, from which other metabolic disturbances associated with obesity are derived. Susceptibility to arterial disease increases with increasing glucose intolerance, and glucose intolerance and plasma insulin are also related to blood pressure[134–136]. Central obesity is associated with an unfavourable plasma lipoprotein pattern – high triglycerides and low HDL cholesterol compared to peripheral obesity. Adipose tissue is a major reservoir of cholesterol, and obese people have an increased cholesterol flux. Garrow has recently summarised the evidence for a primary role of obesity in cardiovascular and other major chronic disease[137].

5.4.5   Treatment of obesity is often difficult and repeated cycles of weight loss and weight gain may be associated with adverse effects[131,132]. Prevention of obesity is therefore particularly important.

5.5   Fetal and infant growth

5.5.1   Recent studies have demonstrated a relationship between growth up to the end of the first year of life and CHD mortality and some of its recognised risk factors in both men and women[138–143]. In particular higher birthweight has been associated with lower blood pressure in middle age[139], and higher weight at one year with improved glucose tolerance[142], and with lower levels of fibrinogen and Factor VII[140] and of apolipoprotein B, the main component of LDL[144].

5.5.2   These observations are consistent with an effect of early development on individuals' later risk of CHD, which may be related to nutritional factors including the method of infant feeding[144]. However it is not clear which, if any, specific nutritional factors are responsible for the observed relationships. The effects on cardiovascular disease mortality seem at least partly mediated through recognised risk factors, and so may help to explain the variation of these risk factors in the population. They appear to act independently of and in addition to contemporaneous environmental effects, such as diet or obesity in later life.

5.6   Diabetes mellitus and insulin

5.6.1   *Diabetes mellitus* is a disorder of carbohydrate metabolism characterised by elevated plasma concentrations of glucose due to insufficient secretion or effectiveness of insulin. It is estimated that there is a two to five fold excess mortality from CHD and stroke in younger diabetics and a two fold excess in older people with diabetes. Peripheral vascular disease is also more prevalent in diabetes. Less severe degrees of glucose intolerance (so called "impaired glucose tolerance") are also associated with increased cardiovascular disease risk[145]. Among diet associated factors, adiposity has consistently been related to increased risk of non-insulin dependent diabetes mellitus (NIDDM), and there is some evidence that diets rich in fat and low in carbohydrate may predispose to this type of diabetes[87,146] (see 5.6.6).

5.6.2   Recently the suggestion has been made that fetal and infantile mal-nutrition may be associated with hypertension, diabetes mellitus and impaired glucose tolerance in later life (see 5.5). Low birth weight and weights at one year of age are associated with higher rates of these conditions in older males[142]. However, there is as yet no evidence linking these variations in growth to maternal, fetal or infantile nutritional status.

5.6.3   *Insulin*   Over the past 25 years there has been recurrent interest in the suggestion that hyperinsulinaemia may contribute to the causation of cardio-vascular disease. It is suggested that insulin increases arterial wall lipid synthesis and smooth muscle cell proliferation. Several epidemiological studies have shown a correlation between insulin levels and cardiovascular disease[147–150] although the associations are not entirely consistent.

5.6.4   Hyperinsulinaemia is found in obesity, in impaired glucose tolerance and in NIDDM, in all of which there is increased risk of cardiovascular disease (CVD). In subjects of normal body weight, the physically fit have lower insulin levels and less CHD then the physically unfit. There is clear evidence of insulin resistance in obesity, impaired glucose tolerance, NIDDM and physically inactive individuals (see 5.9.8). In Asian Indians resident in the UK, who have higher CVD rates than white UK residents, insulin levels are higher. This is consistent with a higher prevalence of diabetes and impaired glucose tolerance as well as central adiposity, higher plasma triglycerides and lower HDL choles-terol[136] (see 5.6.5). High insulin levels are also associated with raised blood pressure. However, although this evidence is suggestive, it is not yet possible to attribute to insulin a specific role in the development of cardiovascular disease.

5.6.5   *Metabolic syndrome (Syndrome X)*   In the last few years increasing attention has been paid to a clustering of cardiovascular disease risk factors – glucose intolerance, hypertension, obesity and dyslipidaemia (raised triglycerides, low HDL cholesterol)[135]. This has been further refined to include central rather than total obesity, physical inactivity and hyperuricaemia[134]. Most of these conditions are also accompanied by insulin resistance. This clustering of risk factors has now been demonstrated in several populations such as Mexican Americans[151], and Hindu and Muslim Indians in North West London, East London, Singapore, Trinidad and Fiji[152]. It is not yet certain whether insulin resistance and consequent hyperinsulinaemia play a causal role in the metabolic syndrome, or whether they are just accompanying facets. The mechanisms whereby insulin resistance could lead to these different conditions is still a matter of debate (see 5.6.3).

5.6.6   There is some, though only, preliminary, evidence to suggest that diets rich in saturated fatty acids might lead to higher plasma insulin levels[153], to insulin resistance and to the development of obesity[154].

5.7   Thrombogenic risk factors

5.7.1   *Normal vascular repair and haemostasis*   The endothelial surface of the blood vessels is subjected to continuous microscopic injury by chemical, biological and mechanical agents. The reparative processes involve many systems, including blood platelets, and the coagulation and fibrinolytic pathways. Receptor proteins on the platelet surface bind to exposed collagen and other glycoproteins, while other platelet receptors bind to fractions released from damaged cells or thrombin generated during coagulation (Figure 5.1). These binding reactions trigger a series of responses which collectively are called platelet activation and comprise:

- shape changes with spreading of the platelet over the damaged surface.

- stimulation of eicosanoid metabolism with production of thromboxane.

- secretion of the contents of platelet storage granules, eg adenosine diphosphate (ADP)

The release of thromboxane and ADP from activated platelets leads to recruitment and aggregation of further platelets at the site of injury.

5.7.2   *Coagulation*   Injury to the vascular endothelium can expose a cell-membrane protein called tissue factor, which combines with the circulating coagulant factor VII. The creation of a tissue factor/factor VII complex initiates a cascade of reactions (the coagulation pathway) which culminates in the generation of thrombin and deposition of an insoluble fibrin network at the site of injury (Figure 5.1). Under normal circumstances the rate of coagulation is regulated by a parallel anticoagulant pathway, but after injury the increased rate of coagulation overwhelms this control. High levels of factor VII activity and of fibrinogen may predispose the blood to clot (a hypercoagulable state), and have been shown to predict CHD independently of each other in middle aged men[155].

5.7.3   *Thrombosis*   More extensive disruption of the vessel wall with breach of the endothelium triggers massive deposition of platelets and fibrin to form a plug to staunch bleeding (thrombosis). This reaction may be large enough to form a haemostatic plug which occludes not only the fissure in the vessel wall, but also the vessel lumen. A thrombotic reaction with potential serious adverse consequences can occur when normal blood is exposed to a highly thrombogenic surface, or when disorders exist in the systems that respond to vascular injury.

5.7.4   *Fibrinolysis*   The fibrinolytic system generates the enzyme plasmin from its circulating precursor plasminogen. Plasmin degrades the insoluble fibrin in clot or thrombus to soluble products (Figure 5.1). Plasminogen is converted to plasmin by the enzyme tissue plasminogen activator (tPA) which is secreted by endothelial cells of the arterial and venous walls. After binding to fibrin, tPA cleaves plasminogen to plasmin, which, in addition to its actions on fibrin, enhances the conversion of plasminogen to plasmin[156]. In this way, fibrinolytic activity is directed to sites of fibrin deposition.

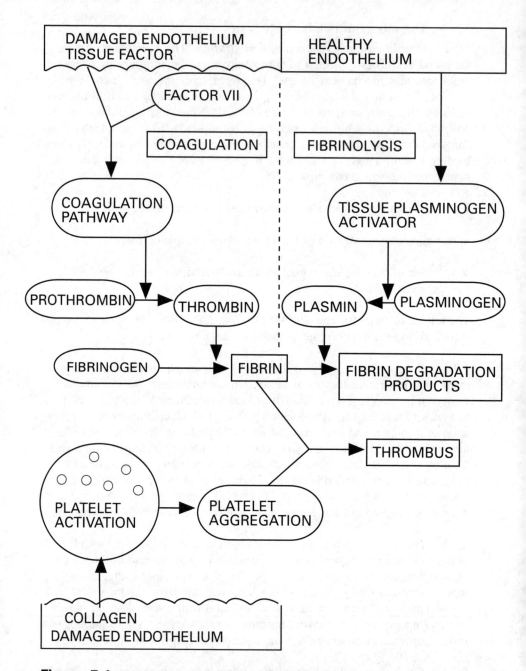

Figure 5.1 *Coagulation follows a cascade of reactions stimulated by a complex of factor VII from the circulation with tissue factor from damaged endothelium. This leads to the formation of an insoluble fibrin mesh. If accompanied by massive platelet deposition due to their activation by exposed collagen, this becomes a thrombus. Fibrinolysis leads to the degradation of insoluble fibrin in a clot or thrombus to soluble products. Under normal circumstances a balance prevents excessive clotting or bleeding.*

118

5.7.5   Fibrinolytic activity is also confined to sites of fibrin deposition by alpha$_2$ – antiplasmin, the circulating inhibitor of free plasmin, and by plasminogen activator inhibitor type 1 (PAI-1) which binds and inactivates tPA, so that the half-life of free tPA in plasma is only a few minutes[157]. Plasma PAI-1 is synthesised by endothelial cells and the liver and is present in platelets. Most plasma PAI-1 circulates in an inactive form that can be activated by binding to a negatively charged surface[158].

5.7.6   Several cross sectional studies have shown an association between measures of low fibrinolytic activity and CHD. Hamsten *et al*[159] found increased PAI-1 in young survivors of a first myocardial infarction who later sustained a re-infarction. Recently, several families have been described in which an inherited elevation in plasma PAI-1 activity is associated with a high risk of thrombosis[160]. A prospective study whose measure of fibrinolytic activity reflected both activation and inhibition of fibrinolysis, found a significant association, after adjusting for fibrinogen, between low fibrinolytic activity and increased risk of CHD in men aged 40–54 at entry which was at least as strong as that for cholesterol[161].

5.7.7   Dietary factors can influence platelet function, and factors in the coagulation and fibrinolytic pathways (see 6.3).

5.8   Smoking

5.8.1   Cigarette smoking is powerfully associated with all forms of acute CHD[162–165], stroke[17,166] including subarachnoid haemorrhage[167], and peripheral vascular disease[168] in both sexes. On average, middle-aged smokers have about double the risk of a major coronary event compared with non-smokers, and heavier smokers are at higher risk[162–164].

5.8.2   The mechanisms by which cigarette smoking promotes CHD are uncertain. Smokers tend to have a more unfavourable diet and plasma lipoprotein pattern than non-smokers, with relatively low HDL cholesterol and high triglyceride concentrations. These latter changes show a dose response relation to the number of cigarettes smoked[169]. Smokers also have a higher plasma fibrinogen concentration than non-smokers[57]; a high plasma fibrinogen has been shown to be a strong predictor of risk of acute coronary events[155,170–172]. Smoking also affects antioxidant status adversely; smokers not only tend to have lower intakes of antioxidant vitamins[173], they also tend to have lower plasma levels for similar dietary intakes[174,175], possibly reflecting a higher turnover of these nutrients. Smokers require higher intakes of vitamin C than non-smokers to maintain similar circulating levels of vitamin C[176]. Cigarette smoking has also been reported to render LDL particles[177] and erythrocytes[178] more susceptible to oxidative modification. The effect on erythrocytes was abolished after supplementation with vitamin E.

5.8.3   Smokers tend to weigh on average several kilograms (2–3 kg) less than non-smokers of similar age, and some gain weight during the first year after quitting[179]. However, the weight gain is not associated with adverse changes in plasma cholesterol, blood pressure and blood glucose[179-181]. Furthermore, plasma HDL cholesterol and apolipoprotein A-I (the major protein of HDL particles) both increase after stopping smoking[182,183] while plasma fibrinogen concentration declines[57]. Many smokers do not gain weight after ceasing to smoke, and most of those who do do not gain excessively. Any adverse effects because of a deterioration in other risk factors are far outweighed by the benefits to health gained by stopping smoking. Weight control can be provided as a component of supervised smoking cessation when required.

5.8.4　Smoking has a particularly adverse effect on cardiovascular disease risk in young women using oral contraceptives. Although the risk of an acute cardiovascular event is very small in pre-menopausal women, individual risk is about 10 times greater in those who smoke and use oral contraceptives than in non-smoking women not using oral contraceptives[184].

5.9　Physical activity

5.9.1　*Introduction*　Physical inactivity is linked to an increased risk of CHD but only a minority of adults takes sufficient exercise to benefit health. To confer benefit, exercise need not be of high intensity. Simple forms of exercise, like walking and cycling, are likely to be effective in decreasing the risk of CHD, and contributing to the maintenance of desirable body weight[29].

5.9.2　*Body fatness*　Exercise has a beneficial effect in the loss of excess body fat[185]. Although the energy expended in walking one mile (just less than 100 kcal or 420kJ) might appear insignificant, the cumulative effects can be major. Even discounting the post-exercise elevation of metabolic rate, the net energy expenditure of walking one mile a day for a year is equivalent to that stored in about 3kg of adipose tissue. The full potential for weight loss applies if there is no increase in energy intake; but fat can be lost despite an increased energy intake. In a well-designed study of a modest programme of jogging, energy intake was stimulated but to a lesser extent than the rise in energy expenditure, resulting in a net loss of body fat[186].

5.9.3　*Weight maintenance*　A gradual increase in physical activity contributes to successful weight loss in obese patients, and individuals who expend about 1500 kcal (6.3 MJ) per week in physical activity tend to maintain their reduced body weight. Habitual low intensity exercise also helps to prevent the common cycle of losing and gaining weight which may incur an additional risk to health (see 5.4). The addition of exercise to a weight reducing regimen increases fat loss and results in greater reduction in the waist to hip ratio[187].

5.9.4　*CHD prevention*　The relative risk of CHD from inactivity appears to be similar in magnitude to that from hypertension, hypercholesterolaemia and smoking[188]. Classic studies found that only those who reported vigorous exercise had a lower risk of fatal and non-fatal heart attacks[189]. For a typical man, this vigorous exercise includes not only vigorous sporting exercise but also fast walking. Men who claimed that their regular speed of walking was fast

(> 4 mph) had a particularly low rate of CHD, and men who walked more than a mile to and from work at a fast pace had a decreased risk compared to other men[190].

5.9.5   A decreased risk of CHD was also evident in Harvard graduates who expended more than 2,000 kcal (8.4 MJ) per week in all types of physical activity (stair climbing, walking and gardening, as well as active sports), regardless of intensity. All causes mortality was 21 per cent lower among men who walked 9 or more miles per week[191]. In the British Regional Heart Study the strength of the inverse relation between physical activity and CHD was not reduced by excluding men who reported doing sporting (vigorous) activity at least once a month[192].

5.9.6   The mechanism by which exercise might help protect against CHD may involve effects on coagulation and thrombosis as well as an influence on lipoprotein metabolism[193]. The lower threshold of exercise needed to modify lipoprotein metabolism (mainly an increase in HDL) appears to be moderate, expending about 1000 kcal (4.2 MJ) per week. The effect is enhanced when the exercise is accompanied by weight loss. Adults who walk for more than two and a half hours per week have more favourable lipid patterns[194,195].

5.9.7   *Blood pressure*   Epidemiological evidence suggests that habitual exercise reduces the risk of arterial hypertension, particularly among those who are overweight[191]. Other studies have found that increasing exercise reduces both the systolic and diastolic pressures of individuals with elevated arterial pressure[196–198], and that these effects are reversed by a return to lower levels of exercise[199]. Comparison of different exercise programmes in hypertensives aged 60–69 years showed that low intensity training can reduce blood pressure at least as much as exercise of moderate intensity[197,200]. Slow calisthenics and stretching exercises do not, however, seem to be effective in this regard and aerobic exercise is necessary[198]. In individuals with hypertension requiring pharmacological therapy, exercise can be a useful adjunct in treatment.

5.9.8   *Insulin sensitivity*   Physical exercise increases insulin sensitivity[201], and may be an effective adjunct to weight reduction in the treatment of non-insulin dependent diabetes mellitus (NIDDM). Middle-aged, well-trained men have lower fasting plasma insulin concentrations and improved insulin sensitivity than untrained men[202]. An inverse relation between energy expenditure in leisure-time activity and the subsequent development of NIDDM has been reported[203]. Habitual physical activity appeared to have the greatest protective effect among men with obesity, hypertension and a parental history of diabetes. Women who take part in regular, vigorous exercise have a lower risk of developing NIDDM[204]. Thus exercise is likely to be effective in the primary prevention of NIDDM as well as in the management of diabetic individuals.

5.9.9   *Effects on blood coagulation and platelet aggregation*   Physical activity has to be continuing and current to confer protection against CHD[190,205]. Exercise might inhibit the clotting process or platelet aggregation (see 5.7).

Plasma fibrinogen concentration is lower in men reporting taking strenuous exercise than in those who do not[206]. An acute bout of exercise is followed by an increase in fibrinolytic activity[207]. Platelet aggregation is also reduced after endurance running[208], although little is known about the effects on platelets of lower intensity exercise.

5.9.10 *Conclusion*   Simple activities like walking, cycling and swimming are effective contributors to reducing CHD risk and maintaining a desirable body weight, and can be modified to suit most age-groups and levels of ability. About 60% of women and 50% of men aged between 16 and 74 do not take regular physical exercise[27]. The potential for reducing morbidity and mortality by changing the exercise habits of the population is therefore considerable.

6.   Diet and risk

Summary

- The likelihood of death from coronary heart disease (CHD) increases with the plasma level of total cholesterol, and particularly of low density lipoprotein (LDL) cholesterol.

- Genetic factors play a part in determining risk of CHD independently of plasma lipid patterns, and may affect individual responsiveness to dietary fats. However for the vast majority of the population the quality and quantity of dietary fat are fundamental and modifiable determinants of plasma lipid levels.

- Plasma cholesterol is significantly influenced by the kinds and amounts of fat in the diet. Fats rich in saturated fatty acids with 12 to 16 carbon atoms raise plasma total and LDL cholesterol, and polyunsaturated fatty acids (PUFA) of the n-6 series lower them. The cholesterol raising effect of the typical dietary mix of saturated fatty acids is about twice as strong as the cholesterol lowering properties of n-6 PUFA. Substitution of saturated fatty acids in the diet with oleic acid, a monounsaturated fatty acid, lowers both total and LDL cholesterol in the plasma.

- High intakes of n-6 PUFA lower HDL cholesterol, an effect not seen with increasing intakes of oleic acid.

- Long chain PUFA of the n-3 series (fish oils) lower plasma triglycerides, and have potentially beneficial anti-thrombotic and anti-inflammatory properties.

- Trans fatty acids, principally from the artificial hydrogenation (hardening) of vegetable and animal fats, raise LDL cholesterol and plasma triglycerides, and lower HDL cholesterol. A positive relationship between trans fatty acid intake, particularly from hydrogenated fats, and risk of CHD has been reported.

- Dietary cholesterol can raise blood total cholesterol, but this effect is less important than that of saturated fatty acids. The response to dietary cholesterol depends on its level in the diet and on the accompanying lipids, and is variable within and between individuals.

- There is a reciprocal relationship between the contributions to food energy of dietary fat and carbohydrate. When starch contributes more than about 60 per cent of food energy blood triglycerides tend to be somewhat higher, and HDL cholesterol lower. However such carbohydrate-rich diets are usually low in saturated fatty acids, and populations consuming them have lower blood LDL cholesterol levels and a lower risk of CHD.

- Diets rich in soluble non-starch polysaccharides (eg from pulses and oats, or in isolated forms such as guar gum) lower post prandial plasma insulin and glucose levels, and LDL cholesterol. Diets rich in non-milk extrinsic sugars tend to raise post prandial plasma insulin, and may adversely affect plasma lipid levels in sensitive individuals.

- Recent studies have reported an inverse association between dietary intake, or blood levels, of antioxidant nutrients and risk of CHD. Antioxidant nutrients (including vitamins E and C, and carotenes) may prevent oxidation of LDL, and this could explain, at least partially, differences in CHD mortality in different populations with similar levels of the major risk factors (intake of saturates and/or plasma total cholesterol, blood pressure and smoking).

- There is good evidence that dietary sodium intake, principally from common salt, is important in determining levels of blood pressure, and in particular the rise in blood pressure with age.

- There is increasing evidence that diets rich in potassium are associated with lower blood pressures and lower risk of stroke. Dietary sources of potassium are widespread. An increase in consumption of fruit and vegetables as recommended would increase dietary potassium intake.

- Blood pressure is raised by excessive consumption of alcohol. Despite this, evidence from a number of studies suggests a protective effect of alcohol consumption on CHD. Alcohol consumption is not recommended as a means of prevention because of the potential for other, adverse, effects.

- Obesity results from chronic energy consumption in excess of expenditure. Obesity in Britain is increasing. Genetic factors as well as low levels of physical activity appear to be important, and interact with dietary factors, in particular the level of fat. Excess fatness is associated with metabolic changes which increase the risk of cardiovascular and other diseases. Although it is possible to consume excess energy from any dietary source, this is more likely the richer the diet is in fat, at least partly because fat is energy dense yet appears to be poor at satiating.

- Restriction of dietary fat is recommended to reduce the likelihood of obesity. In addition restriction of non-milk extrinsic sugars is recommended for those who are, or are becoming, obese.

- Although there is pathological significance in the distribution of body fat there is no known specific dietary determinant of this.

6.1 Introduction

6.1.1 There is a substantial, diverse, and generally consistent body of evidence linking diet and cardiovascular disease[86]. It is derived from laboratory, clinical and population studies, and is most extensive for CHD, in particular for the relationship between CHD and dietary fat. According to this evidence diet influences the risk of cardiovascular disease through its effects on the risk factors for CHD described in Chapter 5, for example blood lipids, and blood pressure, and probably also through thrombogenic mechanisms.

6.1.2 More recent evidence suggests a protective role for dietary antioxidants, such as vitamins E and C and carotenes, possibly through a mechanism which prevents the oxidation of LDL cholesterol.

6.2 Dietary lipids and plasma lipoproteins

6.2.1 Epidemiological and clinical evidence clearly shows that the likelihood of death from CHD is directly related to the level of total cholesterol, and more specifically of LDL cholesterol, in the blood. Reducing elevated plasma LDL cholesterol levels lowers CHD risk (see section 5.2).

6.2.2 Numerous studies have shown that plasma cholesterol levels are significantly influenced by the kinds and amounts of fat in the diet. About 30 years ago, the groups of Keys and Hegsted independently published results of studies of the relationship between fat intake and plasma cholesterol levels[209–211]. They found that, in comparison to carbohydrate, saturated fatty acids in the diet raised plasma cholesterol while polyunsaturated (principally linoleate) fatty acids lowered it. Monounsaturates (principally oleate) were neutral. Equations derived from their work give an indication of the average change in plasma cholesterol in a group of people which could be expected from alterations in the amount and type of dietary fat. Dietary cholesterol was found to have a smaller effect. The equation of Keys et al[210] indicates that the incremental effect of saturated fatty acids on plasma cholesterol is about twice as powerful as the hypocholesterolaemic effect of polyunsaturated fatty acids:

$$\Delta C = 1.35(2\Delta S - \Delta P) + 1.5(\Delta Z)$$

where ΔC = change in serum cholesterol in mg/dl;

ΔS and ΔP = differences between the diets in percentage of calories from saturated and polyunsaturated fatty acids respectively;

ΔZ = difference between the square roots of dietary cholesterol, in mg/1000kcal, of the diets

6.2.3 *Saturated Fatty Acids*   Saturated fatty acids in the diet vary in chain length, the most frequently occurring being palmitic (16:0), stearic (18:0), myristic (14:0) and lauric (12:0). It has been suggested that their cholesterol raising properties result from saturation and suppression of LDL receptors

(See 4.1)[212]. However, not all saturated fatty acids are equally potent in raising plasma cholesterol. Myristic and palmitic are the most effective while stearic acid and fatty acids with 10 or less carbon atoms appear to have no cholesterol elevating effects[210,211,213,214]. The cholesterol response to particular saturated fatty acids may depend in part on the triglyceride structure[215] and in part on LDL receptor activity[216,217]. Both these aspects require further research. The average effect of saturates expressed in the equations of Keys and Hegsted is based on mixtures of saturates as might be found in typical diets. Numerous clinical and other studies over the last 20 years have confirmed these predictions[86,215]. There is no evidence that they are incorrect although mechanisms have not been clearly defined.

6.2.4 *Monounsaturated fatty acids*
6.2.4.1 Early studies indicated that monounsaturated fatty acids, principally oleic acid eg in olive or rapeseed oils lower plasma total cholesterol when they were substituted for saturated fatty acids[209–211]. Enrichment of diets with additional oleate rich fats does not reduce blood cholesterol levels, suggesting that decrements in blood cholesterol come from substitution of monounsaturates for saturates rather than from supplementation alone. Because the effect on plasma total cholesterol is due to the reduction in saturates, mechanistically monounsaturates can be regarded as neutral with respect to plasma total cholesterol. Subsequent work has confirmed the hypocholesterolemic effect of such an exchange both in formula and solid food diets[215].

6.2.4.2 The effect of oleic acid in lowering total cholesterol when substituted for saturates is less than that of linoleic acid[210,211]. Some recent studies, using formula diets, have suggested that the effects of oleic and linoleic acids on LDL cholesterol are similar, and that the greater effect of linoleic acid on total cholesterol is through a reduction of HDL[218,219]. Other studies have suggested that monounsaturated fatty acids have an active LDL cholesterol-lowering effect when substituted for carbohydrates[220–224], although not all studies or analyses are consistent in this respect[215].

6.2.4.3 Linoleic acid incorporated into lipoproteins can increase their susceptibility to oxidation if there is insufficient antioxidant protection[225–227], and may therefore have atherogenic potential[228] (see 3.1). Substitution of saturates by oleic acid would avoid this. Within the limits of total fat intake, substitution of saturates by monounsaturates offers certain theoretical advantages over substitution by polyunsaturated fatty acids. This is consistent with the low incidence of CHD in Mediterranean populations who have traditionally consumed a diet lower in saturates, but richer in olive oil than currently consumed in the UK.

6.2.5 *Polyunsaturated fatty acids*   Polyunsaturated fatty acids are divisible into those of the n-6 and n-3 series (see section 4.1).

6.2.5.1 *n-6 Polyunsaturated fatty acids*   The parent n-6 fatty acid is linoleic acid (C18:2,n-6) which cannot be synthesized in the body and small amounts are essential in the diet (about 2% of dietary energy). Oils from corn, safflower, sunflower and soyabean are rich sources of linoleic acid. When substituted for saturated fatty acids linoleic acid lowers plasma LDL cholesterol (see 6.2.2) and probably also lowers HDL cholesterol, although the latter may be seen only at intakes in excess of about 13% of dietary energy[222].

6.2.5.2 Some but not all population based studies have shown an inverse relationship between adipose tissue linoleic acid (an indicator of long term dietary consumption) and risk of angina pectoris[229] and acute myocardial infarction[230]; and clinical trial data support the view that diets rich in n-6 polyunsaturated fatty acids and low in saturates reduce risk of CHD. However recent work indicates that higher intakes of linoleic acid might result in a higher risk of atherosclerosis[228,231]. Linoleic acid incorporated into lipoproteins is susceptible to oxidation which may lead to modification of the apoprotein. Such an effect in LDL might predispose to the initiation of atherosclerosis (see 3.1, 6.5). There is some concern also that diets rich in n-6 polyunsaturated fatty acids may increase risk of gallstones[232] although this remains uncertain. The possibility that they may promote carcinogenesis in some animal studies remains to be confirmed in human populations[233]. However the safety of average intakes by the population of n-6 polyunsaturated fatty acids in excess of about 6% of energy also remains untested. Consequently diets providing more than about 6% of energy as n-6 polyunsaturated fatty acids cannot currently be recommended.

6.2.5.3 *n-3 Polyunsaturated fatty acids*   The parent molecule, alpha linolenic acid (C18:3, n-3) cannot be synthesized in the body, and is found in green leaves and seeds. The longer chain fatty acids (C:20 and C:22 n-3) are found in oily fish and fish oils. Small amounts of n-3 polyunsaturated fatty acids are essential in the diet of man. Although n-3 fatty acids have a powerful plasma triglyceride reducing action, their effects on LDL and HDL cholesterol are minimal; and when used to treat severe hypertriglyceridaemia, they may increase circulating LDL cholesterol levels. The major effects of fish oils therefore appear to be anti-thrombotic and anti-inflammatory rather than on plasma lipids, though they may also affect the membrane function of some cells (see section 6.3).

6.2.6   *Trans fatty acids*   Hydrogenated fats are a major dietary source of trans and positional isomers of fatty acids (see 4.1.6). More recent 'polyunsaturated' margarines have lower contents of trans fatty acids than older hard margarines. A number of recent expert committees have reviewed the evidence on the biological effects of both kinds of isomeric fatty acid[60,234].

6.2.6.1 The metabolism of trans fatty acids has been recently reviewed by COMA[2], who concluded that trans fatty acids should not be regarded as equivalent either to their cis counterparts or to saturated fatty acids. More recent data on the effects of trans fatty acids on blood cholesterol have since been reported.

6.2.6.2 Investigations of the influence of trans fatty acids on blood cholesterol have shown both elevating and neutral effects, but there are problems in interpretation of much of the data. In 1990 Mensink and Katan[235] published the results of a carefully conducted experiment on 34 women and 24 men in the Netherlands, comparing solid diets with differing contents of oleic (cis C18:1), elaidic (trans C18:1), and saturated (C12-C16) fatty acids. In comparison with oleic acid, C18:1 trans fatty acids were found to raise LDL cholesterol, although not by as much as saturated fatty acids, and to decrease HDL cholesterol. The LDL/HDL cholesterol ratio was higher on the trans fatty acid diet than on the saturated fatty acid diet. The content of trans fatty acids in the experimental diet was relatively high (about 11% of dietary energy, compared to average intakes in the UK of about 2% of energy, although substantially higher intakes might occur in some individuals[60]). A second study using 7% of trans fatty acids found a similar but smaller effect suggesting a linear dose-response relationship[236]. A similar study in Australia, using 7% of energy as elaidic acid, found that elaidic acid raised plasma LDL levels to a similar extent as saturated fatty acids, with no change in HDL levels[237]. A study, conducted by the US Department of Agriculture, substituting either 3% or 6% of energy from oleic acid with trans fatty acids found a dose response rise in plasma LDL cholesterol levels, and a decrease in plasma HDL cholesterol levels at the higher dose of trans fatty acids[238].

6.2.6.3 Findings consistent with those of Mensink and Katan have recently been reported in three epidemiological studies. Troisi et al[239] in a cross sectional study of 748 men found a direct relationship between intake of trans fatty acids and blood total and LDL cholesterol, and an inverse relationship with HDL cholesterol. Willet et al[240] reported findings from the Nurses Health Study, a prospective study involving more than 85,000 women, showing that intake of trans fatty acids was significantly and independently associated with incidence of CHD. The association was seen only for trans fatty acids from hydrogenated vegetable oils. The mainly different trans isomers from ruminant fats did not show such an association. A case-control study in 239 people suffering a first acute myocardial infarction found that after adjustment for age, sex and energy intake, intake of trans fatty acids was directly related to risk of myocardial infarction[241]. Those with the highest intake of trans fatty acids had twice the risk of myocardial infarction as those with the lowest intakes after adjusting for other cardiovascular risk factors. As with the Nurses Health Study, the association was only seen for trans isomers from partially hydrogenated vegetable oils.

6.2.6.4 Two studies have recently been published showing that trans fatty acids at similar levels to those tested above raise Lp(a) levels[237,242]. Mensink et al measured the changes in Lp(a) in three previous experiments comparing 11% and 8% trans fatty acids with saturated fatty acids, monounsaturated fatty acids and linoleic acid. They found that Lp(a) levels were significantly higher on the trans fatty acid diets in comparison with the other diets. They suggested that their previous report that the replacement of the habitual fat by palm oil lowered Lp(a) in normolipidaemic men[243] might have been the result of the displacement of 50% of the trans fatty acids by palm oil. Nestel et al found a significant increase in Lp(a) on a 7% elaidic acid diet compared to a saturated fatty acid diet in mildly hypercholesterolaemic men. A third study, using hydrogenated corn oil, found no effect on Lp(a) levels[244].

6.2.6.5 There are suggestions that trans fatty acids can compete with essential fatty acids, especially at low intakes of the latter, for $\partial 6$ and $\partial 5$ desaturases, the enzymes responsible for converting linoleic acid (C18:2 n-6) and alpha-linolenic acid (C18:3 n-3) to their longer chain derivatives, respectively arachidonic acid (C20:4 n-6) and eicosapentaenoic acid (C20:5 n-3)[245]. Recent research suggests that this might occur even when essential fatty acid intake is not marginal, although this needs to be confirmed[245].

6.2.7 *Dietary cholesterol and plasma cholesterol* The weight of evidence supports the view that raising cholesterol levels in the diet increases plasma cholesterol, primarily LDL cholesterol, although there is considerable inter-individual variation in response. Studies in man over the last 20 years indicate a threshold for an effect at an intake of about 95 mg/1000 kcal (2.5 mmol/1000kcal) with a ceiling at about 450 mg/1000kcal (12 mmol/1000kcal)[65,215]. It is not clear whether the incremental response is linear or curvilinear, at least for cholesterol intakes of less than about 450 mg/1000 kcal (12 mmol/1000 kcal). Excess dietary cholesterol is either not absorbed or suppresses endogenous production. In approximate terms, over the usual range of cholesterol intake in the UK, plasma cholesterol increases by about 0.25 mmol for every 95 mg (2.5 mmol) consumed per 1000 kcal[65,210]. The wide inter-individual variation in response to dietary cholesterol excludes reliable prediction in individuals.

6.2.9 Some studies have found that dietary cholesterol does not influence plasma cholesterol when the diet is low in fat and saturates[246] but not all authors have found this[210] and others have found any interaction to be small[215]. Dietary cholesterol is associated with dietary saturates in usual diets[215] as many of their richer sources are common to both (see 2.3.2) and usual dietary strategies to reduce saturates tend also to reduce dietary cholesterol. However in certain foods, in particular egg yolk, the cholesterol content is disproportionately high compared to the saturates content. The effects of interactions between dietary cholesterol and fat intakes on cardiovascular risk need further investigation. Although the effect on plasma cholesterol of dietary cholesterol is small compared to that of saturates (see 6.2.2), it seems likely that an increase in the dietary concentration of cholesterol from current levels, independent of any change in dietary saturates, would increase plasma cholesterol. There is some evidence that dietary cholesterol may partly influence risk of coronary heart disease independently of its effect on serum cholesterol and this requires further investigation[247]. We therefore recommend that current dietary cholesterol intakes, measured per unit of dietary energy, should not rise.

6.2.10 *Recommendations* We recommend that the average contribution of saturated fatty acids to dietary energy be reduced to no more than about 10 per cent. Monounsaturates (oleic acid) may partly offset this reduction so long as total fat intake does not exceed about 35 per cent of energy (see 6.3 and 6.8). There is reason to be cautious about high intakes of n-6 PUFA and we recommend that the proportion of the population consuming in excess of about 10 per cent of energy should not increase. Trans fatty acid intake in the population should not increase beyond the current estimated average of 5 g/day or 2 per cent of dietary energy and consideration should be given to ways of decreasing the amount present in the diet. The average cholesterol concentration of the diet should not increase.

6.3   Dietary Lipids and Thrombosis

6.3.1   Comparisons between Inuits and Danes and between the inhabitants of a Japanese fishing village and a Japanese farming village found that the higher fish consumers had a reduced tendency for platelet aggregation and a longer bleeding time[248,249]. Other studies have found an inverse relationship between fish consumption and CHD mortality[250,251]. In an intervention trial in men who had already had a heart attack, increasing the consumption of oily fish to two portions a week or consuming the equivalent amount of fish oils resulted in a significant reduction in mortality from CHD and total mortality over the following two years[252].

6.3.2   When the diet is enriched in long chain polyunsaturated fatty acids such as dihomogamma linolenic acid (C20:3n-6) or eicosapentaenoic acid (EPA) (C20:5n-3) from fish oils, they replace arachidonic acid (C20:4 n-6) in membrane phospholipids. In the prostanoid pathway they generate thromboxanes TXA_1 or TXA_3 which are less potent platelet aggregators and vasoconstrictors than the TXA_2 generated from arachidonic acid[253] (see section 5.7). In vascular endothelial cells release of these polyunsaturated fatty acids from membrane phospholipids leads to the production of prostacyclins which inhibit platelet aggregation and are powerful vasodilators[253,254]. Diets rich in fish oils, an abundant source of eicosapentaenoic acid, promote the production of TXA_3, and may reduce platelet aggregation, but do not alter the potency of the endothelial prostacyclins. However, there are only few useful data, in particular those relevant to diet, relating these measures to risk of thrombosis[255,256]. Extrapolation of these experimental findings to the in vivo situation must be made with caution. The effect of dietary fat and fatty acids on the tendency to thrombosis deserves further research.

6.3.3   *n-3 Polyunsaturated fatty acids and platelet behaviour*   Eicosapentaenoic acid in exceptionally large amounts (2.5 g/day or more) can prolong the bleeding time and reduce platelet aggregation[257]. The large amounts of fatty fish needed to achieve these levels of intake of eicosapentaenoic acid (250 g/day or more), as for example in the traditional diet of the Inuit people, are not compatible with the Western diet. Intakes more likely to be acceptable (around 200 g/week) are less likely to produce detectable effects on the platelet or endothelial cell, although physiologically important effects may be undetectable with current techniques. Large amounts of fish oils as dietary supplements increase the urinary excretion of the end-products of metabolism of the prostacyclins, indicating a relative predominance of them over the thromboxanes *in vivo*[258]. However, it is uncertain whether these changes reflect a potentially antithrombotic state at the vessel wall[259,260]. In vitro studies of platelet adhesiveness to segments of arterial wall, fibrinogen or collagen after dietary supplementation with fish oils have produced conflicting results[261,262]. This aspect of platelet behaviour merits further investigation.

6.3.4   *n-6 Polyunsaturated fatty acids and platelet behaviour*   Studies of the effect of dietary linoleic acid (18:2, n-6) on platelet aggregation are conflicting, depending on the agonist employed, the amount of linoleic acid in the diet, and on whether the study was conducted in vivo or in vitro[263,265]. Dietary linoleate has no significant effect on the bleeding time[266].

6.3.5   *Saturated fatty acids and platelet behaviour*   Studies by Renaud have suggested that diets rich in saturates increase platelet aggregability, possibly by increasing platelet and plasma phospholipid content of Mead acid (20:3,n-9), principally derived from stearic acid and a potentiator of platelet aggregation[264,267]. This potentially important effect of dietary stearic acid merits independent investigation.

6.3.6   *Monounsaturated fatty acids and platelet behaviour*   Although oleic acid (18:1, n-9) in the diet appears to displace arachidonic acid in platelet phospholipids, there is little evidence for a significant effect on platelet behaviour or bleeding time[266,268,269].

6.3.7   *Dietary fat and the coagulation pathway*   Factor VII coagulant activity shows an acute increase after a fat-rich meal,and a high factor VII activity is sustained when the diet is habitually rich in fat[270]. These increases can be reversed by a reduction in total fat intake[271,272]. Factor VII coagulant activity has been shown to be a strong predictor of CHD risk in middle-aged men[155]. Fibrinogen levels do not appear to be related to dietary fat intake or fat composition.

6.3.8   Free stearic and palmitic acids, but not unsaturated or short chain saturated fatty acids, increase blood coagulability in vitro[273,274], (see Chapter 5.6). Preliminary short-term feeding experiments have not found an association between dietary fat composition and factor VII activity independent of the effect of total fat[275]. Dietary fish oil supplements appear to have little or no effect on factor VII activity or plasma fibrinogen levels[276-278], but the expression of tissue factor, a component of the coagulant pathway (see 5.6.2), may be reduced by consumption of cod liver oil[279].

6.3.9   *Unsaturated fatty acids and fibrinolysis*   Evidence for an effect of dietary fish oils on plasma tPA levels or the inhibitor of tPA, PAI-1 (see 5.6.4-6) is inconsistent[279-284]. The few available studies of dietary intake of n-6 fatty acids and fibrinolytic activity also gave inconsistent findings[285,286].

6.3.10   *Dietary lipids and blood pressure*   There is some evidence that large doses (3g/day or more) of long chain n-3 fatty acids (EPA and DHA) can induce small reductions in blood pressure in people with mild to moderate hypertension[287,288]. The effects have been less consistent in people with normal blood pressures[288-290]. One trial demonstrated synergism between fish oils and sodium restriction on blood pressure reduction in elderly people[291]. Other unsaturated fatty acids do not appear to have an effect on blood pressure[288].

6.3.11 *Recommendations* Because of their demonstrated clinical benefit in respect of CHD deaths, we recommend an increase in the population's average consumption of long chain n-3 PUFA (principally EPA and DHA) to about 1.5 g/week. This recommendation would be achieved if most of the population consumed fish, especially oily fish, at least weekly. Only about one third of adults consume oily fish weekly, and their intake of long chain n-3 PUFA is 0.27 g/day, or about 2 g/week. In addition consumption of fish would likely substitute for foods more rich in saturates.

6.4   Dietary Carbohydrates

6.4.1   Because there is little variation in the proportion of energy derived from dietary protein, there is a reciprocal relationship between the contributions of dietary fat and carbohydrate to energy. Higher carbohydrate diets are lower in fat, and the metabolic effects of exchanging carbohydrate for fat depend mainly on the degree of the substitution.

6.4.2   Diets where carbohydrate contributes more than about 60 per cent of food energy are associated with higher fasting concentrations of plasma triglyceride, and lower HDL[220,292–294]. Because such diets are low in fat, and usually also in saturates, LDL is also usually low, and populations consuming these diets are characteristically at low risk of CHD. A smaller substitution by carbohydrate to decrease fat from about 40 per cent of energy to about 30 per cent produces only a small rise in fasting triglycerides, and no appreciable fall in HDL[292,295]. There is no evidence that sugars and starches differ in respect of these effects, although the physical (as opposed to chemical) structure of the carbohydrate-containing food may be at least as important.

6.4.3   *Glycaemic index*   There is evidence that both the physical and chemical nature of dietary carbohydrates can influence insulin secretion and postprandial glycaemia. It is possible to rank foods according to their glycaemic index[296], which quantifies the glycaemic excursion following consumption of a standard quantity of the food. However, it is difficult to reproduce this in more complex meals or in whole diets, for which the value of the glycaemic index is not clear.

6.4.4   Diets high in soluble NSP from legumes are associated with lower postprandial insulin and glucose levels. In one long-term population based study[297] glucose levels correlated inversely with legume consumption. There are conflicting data on the impact of high carbohydrate diets on glucose tolerance. Pima Indians on their traditional diet (70% carbohydrate, 15% fat) had lower postglucose insulin levels than when taking a "modern" diet (30% carbohydrate, 50% fat). There is increasing interest in the role of certain starches which, because of their physical and chemical nature, escape digestion in the small intestine to a greater or lesser extent. They then become a quantitatively important substrate for colonic bacterial fermentation similar to NSP.

6.4.5 *Non-starch polysaccharides and serum cholesterol* Oats and beans which contain soluble NSP, and isolated forms of soluble NSP such as guar gum and pectin, selectively lower LDL cholesterol. The amount of NSP used to produce these effects has been substantial compared to usual dietary intakes in many trials, and most of them have been short term studies. A meta-analysis of 10 trials using oatbran or oatmeal found a modest effect on reducing cholesterol levels, depending on the initial levels of cholesterol and the amount of soluble NSP[298]. The average reduction in total cholesterol using 3 g/day soluble fibre from oats was 0.13mmol/L in people with cholesterol levels less than 5.9 mmol/L. Larger reductions were seen in people with higher than average cholesterol levels. Dietary NSP do not appear to affect blood triglycerides or VLDL, and most insoluble forms so far tested do not affect blood cholesterol[2].

6.4.6 *Non-starch polysaccharides and cardiovascular disease* Four prospective studies have shown an inverse relationship between dietary 'fibre' intake and coronary heart disease[9,297,299,300]. The studies have varied in the source of 'fibre' which was to be effective; the trial by Morris et al found that cereal 'fibre' was inversely related to cases of CHD whereas others found that vegetable sources of 'fibre' were associated with decreased risk[9]. A two year intervention trial in men who had already had one heart attack found no effect of increased cereal 'fibre' intake on subsequent risk of mortality from cardiovascular disease[252].

6.5 Antioxidant nutrients and free radicals

6.5.1 The defence of mammalian cells against the detrimental effects of activated oxygen species is a complex process involving a battery of interrelated protective mechanisms. The normal physiological process of reduction of molecular oxygen to water can involve the formation and release of oxygen-derived free radicals. Oxygen free radicals may be important in the aetiology of a number of diseases including some cancers and cardiovascular and cerebrovascular disease. The containment of free radical damage depends on defensive mechanisms, component parts of which are, or are derived from, the micronutrients called 'antioxidants'. These include the essential trace elements selenium, zinc and manganese, and vitamin C and the various forms of vitamin E (the tocopherols and the tocotrienols) of which the natural isomer (RRR) of alpha-tocopherol is the most potent. In addition, beta carotene, and other carotenoids, such as lutein and lycopene (present in large amounts in tomatoes), and flavonoids, present in red wine, tea and onions, probably also play a role.

6.5.2 The addition of electrons to oxygen in its reduction to water results in the formation in sequence of the superoxide anion radical, hydrogen peroxide, and the hydroxyl radical; the most potentially damaging of these is the hydroxyl radical because of its high reactivity with almost any organic molecule. In mammalian cells containing iron the formation of hydroxyl radicals in quantity is probably driven by self-perpetuating iron-catalysed reactions. The accumulation of large amounts of superoxide and hydrogen peroxide is prevented by enzymes that depend on the trace elements mentioned above. Lack of availability of these elements, either for reasons of deficiency in the diet or failure of absorption, might lead to increased generation of hydroxyl radicals.

6.5.3   The targets for hydroxyl radical attack include DNA and proteins as well as the unsaturated fatty acids of lipoproteins and cell membranes. Vitamins E and C, carotenoids, and selenium are all part of the defensive mechanism against lipid oxidation. Lipid peroxyl radicals are quenched by vitamin E, which is located in the surface of lipoprotein molecules. The vitamin E radical so formed is restored to the active form by vitamin C. Lipid hydroperoxides that are formed are removed by selenium-containing enzymes, a vital process because iron can catalyse the formation of further highly reactive lipid radicals.

6.5.4   In summary, there are three lines of defence. The first involves enzymes that depend on trace minerals and prevents the proliferation of oxygen radicals. The second comprises the lipid antioxidants, principally vitamin E, which work together with vitamin C. The third line is the removal of lipid hydroperoxides, catalysed by selenium-containing enzymes.

6.5.5   *Antioxidant nutrients and cardiovascular disease*   Epidemiological studies have found that low plasma levels of vitamins C and E, and diets low in fruit and vegetables, are associated with a higher risk of coronary heart disease. A cross-sectional survey of 1600 middle-aged men in 16 European towns found a significant inverse association between plasma vitamin E concentration and mortality from coronary heart disease[301]. In these populations, differences in plasma vitamin E which ranged from 18 μmol/l to 28 μmol/l explained 62% of the variation in coronary heart disease mortality. A case-control study in Scotland in patients with angina found that plasma concentrations of vitamin E were lower in cases than controls, even after adjusting for smoking[302]. These variations in plasma levels of vitamin E arose from differences in vitamin E consumption in ordinary diets. Two prospective studies in the USA found that the risk of major coronary disease was only significantly reduced in men and women consuming very high levels of vitamin E compared to those consuming the least[303,304]. A significant protective effect was limited to levels of intake only achieved by supplementation (150 mg vitamin E/day). The inconsistency between these studies in the amount of vitamin E associated with reduced CHD risk might be because plasma vitamin E is not only inherently antioxidant but also acts as a marker of a diet with additional antioxidant potential from other dietary constituents, for example carotenoids and flavonoids. There is some evidence that risk of CHD might be affected by consumption of such non-essential but bio-active food components[305]. When taken in isolation, as supplements, higher levels of vitamin E might be necessary to achieve the same effect as the combination of antioxidants present in the sort of diets characterised in the cross-sectional studies.

6.5.6   The peroxidation of polyunsaturated fatty acids in low density lipo-proteins (LDL) is thought to result in the modification of the apoprotein structure of the lipoprotein, forming oxidised LDL. The modified apoprotein is not recognised by the normal LDL receptors on cells but is thought to be taken up instead by 'scavenger' receptors on macrophages[42]. Macrophages can become overladen with oxidised LDL and become foam cells, which may be an early lesion of atherosclerosis. Oxidised LDL has not been measured in vivo but anti-bodies to oxidised LDL can be measured. Men with accelerated atherosclerosis have been found to have had higher levels of antibodies to LDL than controls[306], and men with severe atherosclerosis have been found to have LDL particles which are more susceptible to oxidation than men with less severe atherosclerosis[307].

6.5.7   The susceptibility of LDL to oxidation is affected by a number of factors which include the oxidisability of fatty acids within the LDL particle and the balance of pro- and antioxidants present. LDL particles which contain a larger proportion of polyunsaturated fatty acids are more prone to oxidation in vitro than those which contain higher proportions of monounsaturated fatty acids[225–227,308]. Supplementation with vitamins C and E leads to LDL particles which are less susceptible to oxidation *in vitro*[309,310]. Natural dietary sources of polyunsaturated fatty acids generally contain plentiful vitamin E to protect against oxidation. A comparison of a high polyunsaturated fatty acid diet from sunflower oil with a low fat diet found significantly lower lipid peroxidation on the polyunsaturated fatty acid diet, which was probably due to its higher content of vitamin E[311].

6.5.8   Iron is a pro-oxidant and in its free form can catalyse free radical reactions (see 6.5.2) and has been implicated in lipid peroxidation. Some, but not all, studies have found associations between measures of iron status or iron stores and risk of coronary heart disease and it is still uncertain whether iron status is important in determining CHD risk[312]. High levels of serum ferritin, an iron storage protein and high concentrations of serum iron have been associated with increased risk of coronary heart disease in some studies[313,314] but not in others[315,316]. Low iron-binding capacity was found in one study to be associated with increased risk of myocardial infarction[316] but no association was seen between serum transferrin saturation (serum iron concentration divided by total iron-binding capacity) and risk of coronary heart disease in another study[317]. A 4 year prospective study in the US found that haem iron intake, but not total dietary iron intake, was associated with increased risk of myocardial infarction[318].

6.5.9   *Conclusions*   The evidence for a protective effect of the antioxidant vitamins E and C is persuasive but not yet conclusive[319]. Other substances in foods might be important. Until the results of a number of randomised inter-vention trials currently under way are known, public policy recommendations recommending increased intakes specifically of antioxidant nutrients would be premature. We recommend a diet rich in vegetables and fruit, containing nuts and seeds, and with less saturated oils partly substituting for more saturated fats, which would increase intake of these nutrients and is conducive to general health. The potential risks of purified, high dose supplements in pharmaceutical form are not known. Recent evidence suggests that it would be unwise to assume that they are safe[320]. They are not recommended as a widespread public health policy for CHD prevention.

6.6   Dietary sodium and potassium

6.6.1   Sodium is an essential nutrient, whose balance in the body is maintained by effective homeostatic mechanisms. The intake of sodium in the UK, principally from common salt, exceeds that required to meet metabolic needs[2]. For many years it has been known that in some selectively bred mammalian species the level of blood pressure could be modified by adjusting the salt content of the diet[321]. However, the extent to which this applies to humans has been a matter of controversy.

6.6.2   Numerous studies have shown that in people with blood pressures in the range labelled mild to moderate hypertension, restriction of common salt in the diet reduced blood pressure, in some cases removing the need for anti-hypertensive medication[322–324]. However, evidence that salt restriction reduces blood pressure in the conventionally accepted normal range has been much less uniform[325–327]. This apparent inconsistency in response to salt restriction between two groups who cannot otherwise be distinguished on metabolic criteria led to the suggestion that some individuals, a minority of the population, were constitutionally particularly sensitive to an effect of dietary salt on blood pressure, while in the majority, any such effect was negligible[328]. Dietary salt restriction was seen as an adjunct to conventional treatment in some hypertensive patients, but was not deemed to be an important determinant of prevailing blood pressure levels in the population as a whole. In 1984 COMA concluded that "the dietary intake of common salt should not be increased further and that consideration should be given to ways and means of decreasing it"[1].

6.6.3   Although some populations whose intake of salt was particularly low appear to have a very low prevalence of hypertension, it is not easy to demonstrate such a relationship within single communities. In 1988 the Intersalt Study, a large multinational collaboration, examined the relationship between blood pressure and sodium excretion – a marker of salt intake – in over 10 000 people without clinical hypertension from 52 populations throughout the world[329]. This study demonstrated a positive but weak correlation between sodium excretion and prevailing blood pressure in their populations. A more striking finding was the correlation between sodium excretion and the rise in blood pressure with age. An age related rise in blood pressure is usual in populations such as the UK with moderately high sodium intakes, but virtually absent amongst those with very low sodium diets. In addition, the combination of high sodium excretion, low potassium excretion, high alcohol consumption and obesity appeared particularly predictive of higher blood pressures. More recently the authors have reanalysed their data to take account of statistical bias, and concluded that the relationship between sodium excretion and blood pressure in their study is stronger than previously thought[330].

6.6.4   Unfortunately, in the Intersalt Study it was not possible to say whether the low blood pressures were due to low salt intakes or due to those populations being less urbanized. The populations with the lowest sodium intakes were primitive rural tribes, while those with higher sodium intakes were more urbanized. It remained possible that at least some of the correlation was due to factors other than sodium excretion itself. A meta-analysis by Law et al[331] re-examined data from 24 previous studies around the world, although they did not include the Intersalt data on the grounds that the blood pressures measured in this study were lower than in other studies. Their analysis, which allowed the separation of the effects of urbanisation and of sodium, suggested that both urbanisation and sodium have independent effects throughout the range of observed blood pressures. The relationship observed in this analysis was considerably stronger than that seen in the Intersalt study. Furthermore, based on the relationship seen in the observational studies, Law et al were able to predict the reduction seen in clinical studies of sodium restriction.

6.6.5   Law et al suggested that there was a quantifiable and predictable effect of sodium restriction on blood pressure in clinical studies, consistent with that observed between populations, so long as the studies had continued for long enough to allow the sodium restriction to exert its effect, at least five weeks[331]. The effect on blood pressure depended on the degree of sodium restriction, and was higher in older people and in those with higher initial blood pressures. Their analysis has been criticised[332] on the grounds that the size of the effect was due to the inclusion of non-randomised studies which could not exclude an artefactual or placebo effect. If these studies are excluded the effect on blood pressure is considerably less. However, many of the remaining randomised studies were on younger people with only mild hypertension, in whom, according to the observations of Law et al, the blood pressure reduction would be expected to be less than in older people with higher initial blood pressures[333]. Based on their data and the average age of the English population[27], an average reduction in systolic blood pressure of about 3.5mm Hg would be expected to result from an average reduction in sodium of 50mmol/day[331].

6.6.6   Although common salt, sodium chloride, is the major source of sodium in the diet, there are others, eg sodium acetate or bicarbonate. In clinical studies, the effect of sodium chloride on blood pressure has been shown to exceed that of other sodium salts[328]. The possibility also exists that the chloride ion may be responsible for the observed effects. However a substantial proportion of chloride in the diet is derived from many other sources than common salt and it therefore seems unlikely that the above relationships can be ascribed to chloride alone. Nevertheless the combination of sodium and chloride appears particularly prone to affect blood pressure.

6.6.7   In contrast to sodium, higher dietary potassium intake may reduce blood pressure. Although the evidence for this is less than that relating to sodium and blood pressure, a recent meta-analysis of the data confirmed such an effect, which was greater the longer the period of potassium supplementation, and the higher the initial blood pressure[334].

6.6.8   *Conclusions*   Sodium intake appears to be an important determinant of blood pressure in the population as a whole at least partly by influencing the rise in blood pressure with age. Although the quantitative degree of sensitivity to salt is still unclear, it appears to be greater with increasing age and higher initial blood pressure, and contributes to the quantitatively more important effects of obesity and alcohol intake. A diet lower in common salt and higher in potassium would be expected to result in lower blood pressure and to a smaller rise in BP with age.

6.6.9   The predominant source of salt in the UK diet is manufactured foods (estimated at about 65–85% of the total[4,335]). Therefore while some reduction of salt intake can be made by reducing salt in cooking or added at the table, at least as great a potential effect would be possible from reducing the salt content of manufactured foods. For instance an average slice of bread may contain 0.4 g salt (0.16 g sodium). Potassium is a component of many foods, and vegetables and fruit, eg tomatoes, and some manufactured foods and drinks are rich sources (see 2.3.3.9). The possibility, including the safety, efficacy and acceptability, of substituting potassium chloride for sodium chloride in bread should be explored, as this might prove a useful and practical way of reducing the sodium content of this food[336]. In addition an increase in potassium intakes resulting from this exercise might be valuable.

6.6.10   *Recommendations*   In order to reduce the population's average blood pressure (and particularly the rise in BP with age), as well as the numbers of people requiring antihypertensive medication or at high risk of CHD and stroke, the diet should contain less sodium, principally from common salt, and more potassium, principally from vegetables and fruits. An average reduction of 50 mmol sodium/day (3 g salt/day), has been estimated to result in an average reduction in systolic blood pressure of about 3.5 mm Hg[331]. A larger effect would be likely to be seen over the longer term as the rise in blood pressure with age was also reduced. We recommend a gradual reduction in average sodium intake by the adult population to about 100 mmol/day (6 g salt/day), and an increase in potassium intake to about 90 mmol/day (3.5 g/day). It is expected that intakes by adults will exceed those by children, and that those by men will be greater than those by women. Research should be conducted into effective means of implementing this recommendation.

6.7   **Alcohol**

6.7.1   The consumption of alcohol in sensible quantities and in appropriate circumstances provides many people with enjoyment; however, alcohol is also linked to morbidity, mortality and social problems. In 1986 the cost of alcohol-associated illness in Britain was estimated at £167 million[337] and the overall social cost is now around £2.5 billion[338]. While there is no dispute that heavy alcohol consumption is associated with increased mortality, abstainers have also been found to have increased risk, and this relationship between alcohol consumption and mortality, the so-called U-shaped curve, has been the subject of much debate[339].

6.7.2   The levels of consumption of alcohol recommended by the medical profession as unlikely to cause harm to health are 14 units weekly for women and 21 units weekly for men[340]. One unit is defined as the equivalent of 8 g pure ethanol. These levels are based on a number of considerations, biological, psychiatric and social, but did not take into account possible protection from CHD (see 6.7.7).

6.7.3   *Alcohol and blood pressure*   A number of studies have shown a relation between alcohol consumption and blood pressure[341–343]. The INTERSALT study found that men who were non-drinkers had systolic blood pressures 2.7 mmHg lower than consumers of 300–499 ml (about 30–50 units) alcohol per week and 4.6 mm Hg lower than consumers of 500 ml or more, independent of age[329]. Findings in women were similar.

6.7.4   Although blood pressure rises with acute alcohol consumption, it is also related to habitual consumption, particularly at higher intakes in excess of about 300 ml alcohol weekly (about 30 units weekly, or four "standard" drinks daily).

6.7.5   *Alcohol and stroke*   Both acute and habitual heavy alcohol consumption increase risk of stroke, particularly cerebral haemorrhage (see 3.4)[344,345]. Moderate alcohol consumption may increase risk of haemorrhagic stroke, but in the Nurses Health Study overall risk of stroke was lower in moderate consumers of alcohol[346].

6.7.6   *Alcohol and CHD*   There is a strong inverse association between national average wine consumption and national CHD mortality[347]. Longitudinal studies demonstrate higher total mortality in heavy drinkers, but predominantly due to causes other than CHD[348]. Alcohol consumption appears consistently to be associated with relatively low risk of CHD across a variety of studies in diverse populations[6]. In the US Nurses Health Study, and the Health Professionals Follow Up Study, alcohol intake was associated with a substantial reduction in risk of CHD[346,349]. The addition of alcohol consumption to regression analysis of CHD risk factors decreases the unexplained variance[350].

6.7.7   The interpretation of the higher CHD risk in non drinkers is complicated because non-drinkers include people who have given up drinking because they were unwell[351]. Such people would be expected to have higher rates of disease, and their inclusion with the non-drinkers might account for the high CHD rates found in non-drinking groups and many studies had information only on current rather than lifetime drinking habits. However, where such information was available, those who had never drunk alcohol also had higher CHD mortality than drinkers[348,349,352–357]. Ex-drinkers who stop for medical reasons appear to have higher risk confined to non-cardiovascular mortality[353].

6.7.8   Alcohol consumption is associated with increased levels of HDL cholesterol[358,359] which are associated with reduced CHD risk (see section 5.2). About half the association between non-drinking and CHD can be accounted for statistically by lower levels of HDL cholesterol[355,360]. Alcohol consumption is also associated with lower levels of plasma fibrinogen[361] and with reduced platelet activity, and hence with a lower probability of thrombosis[362] (see section 5.7).

6.7.9   Some alcoholic beverages contain bioactive components other than alcohol. In particular, red wine contains polyphenols (a kind of flavonoid) which are antioxidants and capable of inhibiting LDL oxidation in vitro (see 6.5)[363]. Consumption of alcoholic drinks containing these compounds may contribute to the lower CHD risk in light drinkers.

6.7.10   Alcohol can adversely affect cardiovascular disease through its effect in raising blood pressure at intakes above about 4 units of alcohol (35 g) a day. This could, in part, account for the increased risk of stroke. At higher levels, alcohol is associated with cardiomyopathy. At two units (about 16 g) alcohol a day there may be no cardiovascular harm and some degree of protection from CHD with some net benefit for those at risk from this condition (men aged over 35 and post-menopausal women). Above three units a day there is good evidence of increasing biological risk as well as social harm. There appears to be a strong association between the average levels of alcohol consumption in a population and the prevalence of heavy drinking[364], though this has not always been accepted[365]. Hence an increase in the mean level of consumption may well denote an increased prevalence of heavy drinking. The balance of risk and benefit is against recommending the public to consume alcohol to lessen the risk of CHD[337].

6.8   **Diet and obesity**

6.8.1   Excess fatness in adults causes metabolic changes which increase risk of cardiovascular and other diseases (see section 5.4). As with many biological variables, the development of obesity results from the interaction of environmental and genetic factors, but inevitably follows chronic energy consumption in excess of expenditure[366]. The distribution of body fat is also important in determining cardiovascular risk, but there is no known dietary determinant of this.

6.8.2   Around the world certain populations appear particularly prone to develop obesity when in an environment which permits it. For instance amongst the Pima Indians of Arizona exposed to a typical Western diet approximately half the adult population is obese[367]. Similarly, within populations, obesity clusters in certain families. A proportion of this concordance is genetic, but common

140

environmental factors also play a part. Not all individuals, even identical twins, have the same propensity to become fat. Identification of susceptible individuals would be valuable, but there are many constitutional factors which combine to determine individual susceptibility; these are as yet incompletely understood and difficult or impractical to measure. Non genetic factors are therefore important, especially since they can be modified.

6.8.3   Factors affecting energy expenditure include basal metabolic rate, voluntary and other physical activity and dietary induced thermogenesis. Of these, only voluntary physical activity can be substantially modified by individuals. Moderately precise and accurate methods of measurement exist for at least some of these factors, and for total energy expenditure. Measurement of habitual dietary energy intake is less easy to ascertain, and all methods are known to be subject to certain biases. There are few data on dietary energy intake in relation to the development of obesity, as most studies have addressed the diets of people already obese, rather than the pre-obese. Cross sectional epidemiological studies have generally observed an inverse relationship between energy intake and measures of body fatness[368-370]. This is likely to reflect, at least partly, higher energy intakes in the more physically active. In the study by Romieu et al, the association disappeared when controlled for age and exercise[368]. In general basal metabolic rate is higher in obese people because they have higher lean body mass as well as fat[2].

6.8.4   Diets relatively high in fat and low in carbohydrate are more energy dense than low fat diets and might therefore be more conducive to the development of obesity. In addition, in situations of positive energy balance, the conversion of excess energy as carbohydrate to adipose tissue requires more energy than the conversion of excess energy from dietary fat[371]. Cross-sectional studies have observed a positive correlation between the proportion of dietary energy as fat and measures of body fatness[368,372]. It has been reported that, at least in the short term, people spontaneously eat more calories and gain weight when offered a high fat diet compared to a medium fat diet[373]. On a low fat diet these subjects spontaneously ate 627 kcal/day less energy and lost weight. The subjects also ate 84 g/day more food than on the high fat diet, indicating a small amount of caloric compensation. Other studies have shown that physical activity is more likely to lead to weight loss when combined with a low fat diet (20% energy) than with higher fat diets (40–60% energy)[374-6].

6.8.5   There is mounting and persuasive evidence that fat has less satiating effect than carbohydrate. Control of energy intake can be described in two main ways. The constraint on meal size is described as satiation, while the reluctance to start eating is called satiety. Their determinants are not necessarily identical. In obese women, both hunger and the fat content of a meal increase energy intake at that meal but have little effect on subsequent energy intake[377]. This implies that dietary fat has only weak effects both on satiation (stopping eating) and on satiety (not starting to eat). These relatively weak effects combine with the relatively high energy density of fat-rich diets to increase the likelihood of eating a diet containing excess energy, so-called passive over-consumption of calories[378].

6.8.6   For protein and carbohydrate, mechanisms exist to maintain day to day balance within quite narrow limits, and different priorities exist within the body for the oxidation of macronutrients, with fat lowest in the hierarchy[379]. Chronic overconsumption of protein and carbohydrate, and of alcohol, therefore lead to weight gain by diverting dietary fat from metabolism to storage. The hypothesis has been proposed that the need to maintain carbohydrate stores is an important determinant of voluntary food intake and, therefore, that high fat diets lead to increased energy intakes in order to meet the requirement for carbohydrate[380]. However, other studies have not found that glycogen stores, *per se*, affect food intake in humans[381]. Research into the effects of dietary composition on the propensity to obesity should be pursued. More information is also needed on the effect of interactions between diet and body fatness on risk.

6.8.7   *Conclusions*   Taken together, these observations strongly suggest that a high fat diet facilitates passive overconsumption of energy and weight gain, particularly in situations of low physical activity. Treatment of established obesity is notoriously difficult. Prevention of obesity is therefore important, but identification of susceptible individuals is insufficiently precise. The risk of developing obesity depends on exposure to an environment conducive to excess energy consumption, ie a diet rich in fat, combined with low levels of energy expenditure. Although it is possible to consume excess energy from any dietary source, it is rendered more likely the richer the diet is in fat. The fat content of the UK diet along with other westernised societies is high. Controlled clinical studies of reduced dietary fat intake in established obesity are conflicting, but usual clinical practice involves the prescription of low fat diets[366]. It is likely that reduced dietary fat will over time also lead to reduced occurrence of obesity. Reduced total energy intake can sensibly be aided by the avoidance of non-milk extrinsic sugars (which often occur in foods in combination with fat), since such avoidance does not imply lower intakes of other, valuable, nutrients. Such measures are widely accepted as the most appropriate dietary strategies for the treatment of established obesity[366].

6.8.8   We recommend that, in order to reduce the likelihood of obesity in the population, the average consumption of total fat as a proportion of energy should be reduced. We consider the target of about 35% of energy to be a significant reduction which is potentially achievable. Strategies to reduce the occurrence of obesity should include promotion of physical activity. In addition, non-milk extrinsic sugars consumption should be restricted in those who are or are becoming obese. Research should be carried out to determine effective and acceptable ways of implementing this recommendation and to define further the nature of the relationship between dietary factors, including fat consumption, and obesity.

6.9   Miscellaneous factors

6.9.1   *Hardness of water*

6.9.1.1 A weak inverse association between water hardness and cardiovascular disease mortality has been reported in a number of studies. The size of the effect is small and the relationship is most clearly seen at water hardness levels below 170 mg/l (as $CaCo_3$). Increases in water hardness above this level are not associated with further reductions in mortality. In 1974, the COMA Panel on Diet and Cardiovascular Disease advised caution on proposals to soften water supplies[18], and in its 1984 report, noted that an EEC Directive, due to be implemented in 1985, would require a minimum hardness for water which had been artificially softened[1]. The 1984 Panel commented that "Individual members of the public who soften water in their own homes may wish to take the precaution of drinking unsoftened water."[1]

6.9.1.2 Since 1981 further studies have not altered the balance of the evidence and the explanation for the association remains unknown. Nevertheless in view of the consistency of the evidence it remains prudent not to undertake softening of drinking water supplies.

6.9.2   *Coffee*

For over 20 years it has been suspected that caffeine or coffee consumption may contribute to the development of CHD[382], but the evidence remains inconsistent[383–385]. There is little evidence that caffeine itself has any relation with CHD risk, but there are other components of coffee which might partly account for some observed associations. The Scandinavian practice of boiling coffee during its preparation appears to generate a hyper-cholesterolaemic fraction[386,387], but the relevance of this to the UK population is unclear. Coffee drinking as practised in the UK does not appear to affect CHD risk[388].

6.9.3   *Tea*

Tea drinkers have similar caffeine intakes to coffee drinkers, but there is little evidence for any effect of tea consumption on plasma cholesterol or CHD[388]. Recently the suggestion has been made that tea, a rich source of antioxidant flavonoids (see 6.5.1), might protect against CHD, at least in older people[305], but these data need replication.

6.9.4   *Homocysteine*

Individuals who are homozygous for the autosomal recessive condition homocystinuria have high blood levels of the amino acid homocysteine, and are at increased risk of premature cardiovascular disease[389]. Homocysteine is a highly reactive amino acid which can be directly toxic to vascular endothelium, potentiate oxidation of LDL and promote thrombosis. There is some evidence that blood homocysteine levels below those found in homocystinuria might contribute to cardiovascular risk[389], but the relevance of this to the population at large is not known. Vitamin B_{12} and folate are involved in the metabolism of homocysteine but there is currently no evidence that intakes of these vitamins influence risk of cardiovascular disease[390].

6.9.5   *Garlic and onions*

Garlic has been advocated as a remedy for a variety of ills for centuries. The principal bioactive ingredient is alliin, which on disruption of cloves is converted to allicin. The bioactive ingredients cause the characteristic odour, which can be masked in preparations, but apparently not in consumers. Natural concentrations of allicin can vary tenfold, although there is some standardisation of commercial preparations. Onions contain smaller amounts of alliin, but also contain significant concentrations of antioxidant flavonoids, such as quercetin (see 6.5.1), which might have potential to influence atherogenesis. There is only a small amount of good data on the biological effects of garlic, not all of which is consistent. Large doses – over 7 cloves daily - appear to be necessary for any effects, which are reported to include inhibition of platelet aggregation, increase in fibrinolysis, reduction in plasma concentrations of fibrinogen, and of total and LDL cholesterol, and an increase in HDL cholesterol. There is no evidence for an effect on clinical events either of fresh garlic or onions, or of commercial preparations[391,392].

7. Children

Summary

- A number of processes linked with the development of atherosclerosis have their origins in childhood, but the degree to which this determines the occurrence of atherosclerosis in adulthood is unclear.

- The growth of the fetus and infant, and possibly therefore their diets and those of the mother before and during pregnancy, may be implicated in the development of cardiovascular disease in adult life.

- Those individuals with blood lipids, blood pressure and body mass index in the higher reaches of the distribution in childhood are likely to remain in the upper reaches during adulthood.

- The dietary and other recommendations in this report do not apply before the age of 2 years, but apply in full from the age of 5 years. A flexible approach is recommended to the timing and extent of dietary change for individual children between the ages of 2 and 5 years.

7.1   The extent to which atherosclerosis has its onset during childhood is a matter of controversy[393]. Fatty streaks, which some have regarded as precursors of atheromatous plaques, are present from early childhood. However streaks occur equally in populations with a high risk of vascular disease and in those with a low risk[394]. Fatty streaks are reversible and may be a response to a transient fat load rather than progenitors of vascular disease, although they might indicate susceptible sites for future atheroma. True atheromatous plaques first appear in otherwise normal children around the time of puberty, and are more common in white than in black children in Western countries[395]. Fatty streaks may therefore be a necessary though not sufficient precondition for atherosclerosis (see chapter 3).

7.2   A number of epidemiological studies, in different populations[396–8], have demonstrated tracking of CHD risk factors (plasma lipids, blood pressure and obesity) from around 2 years of age into adult life. Forty per cent of children with cholesterol in the highest quarter of the distribution can be expected to maintain this position in adult life. About ninety per cent of young adults with plasma cholesterol of 240 mg/dl (6.2 mmol/l) or more[399] might be identified in childhood, either by plasma cholesterol above the upper quartile or by the presence of obesity. Although no comparable studies have been made in the UK, and child rearing practices undoubtedly differ between different societies, it is reasonable for children of school age to adopt the dietary patterns recommended for lower plasma cholesterol in the adult population.

7.3   Early growth and development appear to be important determinants of individual constitutional susceptibility to cardiovascular disease and some of its risk factors. Recent studies have demonstrated a relationship between growth up to the first year of life and CHD mortality and some of its risk factors in both men and women[138,143] (see 5.5).

7.4   *Infants' diets (under 1 year)*   There is no doubt about the health benefits of breast-feeding during early infancy and a continued intake of breast-milk or infant formula continues to be recommended throughout the first year[400]. The average fat content of milk from well-nourished mothers is about 4.2 g/100 ml (about 55 per cent of energy). There is considerable variability in this figure which appears to be diet related, and in affluent countries it may reach 60 per cent, while in poor countries it may be no more than 40 per cent; the energy deficit is off-set by higher concentrations of lactose[401]. The fatty acid composition of breast milk reflects the mother's dietary intake. Thus the milk from women on a Western-type diet has palmitic (C16:0) and oleic (C18:1, n-9) as the principal fatty acids with lauric (C12:0), myristic (C14:0), stearic (C18:0) and linoleic acids (C18:2, n-6) in smaller quantities. Polyunsaturated fatty acids contribute 2 per cent of the total energy[402]. Cholesterol is present at a level of about 16 mg per 100 ml[403]. Changes in the diets of pregnant and lactating mothers are likely to affect the intake of the breastfed infant.

7.4.1   Neither breast-milk nor infant formula can supply all the nutritional needs of the infant during the second six months of life. Weaning foods should contribute to the energy and nutrient intake as well as starting to provide the diversity of textures and tastes that are a part of normal development. An expert COMA working group on weaning and the weaning diet is presently examining this important aspect of infant feeding.

7.5   *The diets of children aged one to five years*   The amount and nature of the fat currently eaten by pre-school children in the UK and the proportion of the total energy it contributes are not known. A programme of national diet and nutrition surveys, jointly commissioned by the Department of Health and Ministry of Agriculture, Fisheries and Food has recently examined the eating patterns and nutritional status of children aged 1½ to 4½ years and results are expected in 1994. Based on earlier surveys[404], it is likely that the mean proportion of food energy derived from fat by very young children in the UK is about 40 per cent. Therefore, if the target of about 35 per cent of energy from fat is to be achieved by the age of 5 years, there will need to be a reduction in the fat content of the diet by this age. The best way of achieving this reduction must take account of the nutritional, physiological and psychological needs of children under five and is likely to vary from child to child, from family to family, and from culture to culture. It is especially important that growth is not compromised through provision of inappropriately bulky and low energy diets.

7.5.1   *The diets of children aged 1 to 3 years*   Between the ages of 1 and 3 years toddlers are rapidly learning new skills. They develop new tastes, likes and dislikes and many manipulate food intake as a way of obtaining parental attention. They may pass through periods in which a few food items can seem to be the major contributors to maintaining energy intake and the diet appears to be very restricted. Advising against individual foods simply because they may be perceived as contributing too much fat will reduce the parents' options for diversifying and may even imperil the nutritional adequacy of the diet. There is no evidence that passing and individual food fads are carried through to adult life from this early period[405]. In view of the overriding importance of adequate intake, these short term preferences should not be considered nutritionally detrimental.

7.5.2 *The child's diet at 4 years* By the age of 4 years many children are taking some meals with the family. The dietary recommendations for adults could therefore influence the children's intake and this is appropriate, provided that energy intake is sufficient and growth satisfactory. Snacks may be required to promote diversity in the diet and to contribute to energy and nutrient intakes.

7.6 *The diets of schoolchildren* The diets of schoolchildren, in terms of their nutrient balance, are similar to the rest of the population. There is little information on the long-term effects of diet in children of school age and limited information on factors which affect childrens' food choices. In 1984 COMA advised that children aged 5 years and above should moderate their dietary fat intake along with the rest of the population[1], and this approach has received general endorsement. The present recommendations are likewise applicable from 5 years onwards throughout childhood.

7.7 *Milk in the diet* In many Western countries whole cows' milk is an important item in the diet of pre-school children over 1 year and contributes especially to energy, calcium, protein, and micronutrient intakes. Any reduction in the intake of whole milk by such children in the UK, unaccompanied by substantial compensatory changes in the rest of the diet, might therefore have undesirable effects on their nutritional status and growth.

7.7.1 Fully skimmed cows' milk has lower energy, fat and vitamin A content than whole milk. It is therefore not suitable as a staple food in an otherwise conventional diet for children under the age of 5 years. Semi-skimmed cows' milk has a fat content of 1.6 g/100 ml compared to 3.8 g/100 ml in whole milk, but for the same reasons is unsuitable as a main drink below the age of 2 years under normal circumstances.

7.7.2 Limited experience from Canada and Sweden[406,407] indicates that introducing semi-skimmed milk into the diet of 2 year olds can have no adverse effect on growth. Similar studies have, however, not been done in the UK. Nevertheless, for children who are consuming a diverse diet and who are growing well, the introduction of semi-skimmed milk should be possible from the age of 2 years without harm although it is uncertain whether it will influence the future health of the child. Parents in families where semi-skimmed milk is generally consumed may choose this or switching from whole to semi-skimmed milk could be delayed until nearer the fifth birthday.

7.8   *Other foods and nutrients*   A reduction in the contribution of fat to dietary energy intake should be compensated by an appropriate increase in starchy foods such as bread, potatoes, rice and pasta, and these foods should increasingly contribute to the total energy intake as the child approaches school age. Foods high in NSP should not be emphasised unduly in this age group at the expense of more energy rich foods required for growth; in particular foods rich in cereal fibre such as wholemeal bread should not be pressed on young children who may prefer other types of bread. Vegetables and fruit should be encouraged where possible.

7.9   No salt should be added to baby food or foods specifically marketed for young children. There is evidence of the benefit to health of lower salt diets for the population as a whole[331], and a lower intake can safely be recommended for all children.

7.10   *Conclusions*   Children between the ages of 1 and 5 years are at their most individualistic. This applies especially to their behavioural, social and cultural maturation. Firm age related targets for eating practices are unrealistic. These flexible guidelines within a year by year schema offer a good chance of achieving the recommendations – that by the age of 5 years children should consume a diet which on average contains no more than about 35 per cent of the calories from fat and about 10 per cent of the calories from saturated fatty acids.

7.11   *Recommendations*   We recommend that by the age of 5 years children should be consuming a diet based on the recommendations for adults in this Report. Research should be carried out into the definition of optimal growth for children in relation both to their current and future health; into how nutritional factors contribute to optimal growth and into the nutritional determinants of differences in growth between groups of children in the UK.

8.   Older People

Summary

- CHD and stroke rates rise sharply after the age of 65 years and are the leading causes of death and serious illness among older people. The number of people over this age is expected to rise by about a quarter in the next 30 years.

- There is evidence that lifelong diet is important in maintaining good health in older people, although more data are needed on the relationships between current diet and cardiovascular disease at this stage of life.

- Recent declines in rates of cardiovascular mortality have occurred in older age groups as well as in younger ones, and in both sexes.

- The recommendations in this Report apply in general to all adults, but special care is needed as people get older to avoid diets inadequate in energy and nutrients if inappropriately stringent dietary advice is followed. The maintenance of moderate levels of physical activity, and an increase in the consumption of fruit, vegetables and fish are of particular importance.

8.1   The annual incidence of cardiovascular disease, predominantly CHD and stroke, increases exponentially with increasing age from around 200 per 100 000 in men aged 50–54 to around 2500 per 100 000 in men aged 80–84, and is the leading cause of mortality in older people. It is also a major cause of morbidity and results in long-term disability and dependency. The proportion of the total population in England and Wales aged 65 years and over is now 16 per cent, or approximately 7.8 million persons. It is projected to increase to 20 per cent, or 9 million persons, by 2020.

8.2   Much of the scientific evidence on which current dietary recommendations for the prevention of cardiovascular disease are based comes from studies in middle-aged men and it is not yet certain how they apply to older people of both sexes. More information is needed on the relationship between diet and cardiovascular disease in elderly people, particularly elderly women. Some studies have shown relationships between dietary intake and subsequent cardiovascular disease in older people, although there is currently little evidence in this age group on the effects of changes in diet. Prospective studies indicate that in older persons up to 80 years of age blood cholesterol and blood pressure continue to predict CHD but less strongly than in younger people[408–413]. The relationship is less strong and less consistent in older women than in older men[412]. An analysis of the prospective studies by Law *et al* (1994) showed that a reduction in cholesterol concentration in men of 0.6 mmol/l was associated with a reduction in risk of 54% at age 40, 20% at age 70 and 19% at age 80[12]. However although the *relative* risks associated with higher levels of these risk factors are less than in younger people, the reduction in *absolute* risk is substantial because mortality rates are higher in older people[413]. The potential for benefit is therefore great.

8.3   In the USA the reduction in CHD risk factors in the population explains at least partly the large decline in CHD mortality in all age groups of adults. Further reductions in the occurrence of disease and disability in the elderly could also be expected from improvements in health at younger ages.

8.4   Until trial data on the effects of dietary change in the elderly are available, decisions about whether, and if so which, recommendations are warranted need to be based solely on judgements about potential benefits and risks. We endorse the recommendation of the COMA Report on the Nutrition of Elderly People that elderly people should be encouraged to adopt diets which moderate their plasma cholesterol levels[414] because of the potential benefit in the reduction of absolute risk. Recommendations for increases in vegetable, fruit and fish consumption are dietetically appropriate, and may be especially valuable, for older people. They may have considerable benefits not just for prevention of cardiovascular disease but for other chronic diseases and quality of life. There is sufficient evidence that moderate physical activity in later life such as walking is a valuable contributor to general health, and that reduction in salt intake at this age may be particularly effective in lowering blood pressure. We recommend increased consumption of fruits and vegetables, and fish, and the maintenance of moderate levels of physical activity, such as walking.

8.5   Diet is an important determinant of good health in older people. The Review Group agreed that the recommendations in this Report apply to all healthy adults including most elderly people. However it is particularly important for some older people to avoid energy and nutrient deficiencies from inappropriately stringent dietary advice especially those who have conditions which limit the relevance and practicality of these recommendations. Adequate energy intake is paramount, and advice which may compromise this in people with poor appetites should be avoided.

9. References

[1] Department of Health and Social Security. *Diet and Cardiovascular Disease: Report of the Panel on Diet in Relation to Cardiovascular Disease, Committee on Medical Aspects of Food Policy*. London: HMSO, 1984. (Report on Health and Social Subjects; 28).

[2] Department of Health. *Dietary reference values for food energy and nutrients for the United Kingdom: Report of the Panel on Dietary Reference Values, Committee on Medical Aspects of Food Policy*. London: HMSO, 1991. (Report on Health and Social Subjects; 41).

[3] Ornish D, Brown SE, Scherwitz LW *et al*. Can lifestyle changes reverse coronary heart disease? *Lancet* 1990; **336**: 129–33.

[4] Gregory J, Foster K, Tyler H, Wiseman M. *The dietary and nutritional survey of British adults: a survey of the dietary behaviour, nutritional status and blood pressure of adults aged 16 to 64 living in Great Britain*. Office of Population Census and Surveys. Social Survey Division. London: HMSO, 1990.

[5] Marmot MG, Syme SL, Kagan A, Kato H, Cohen JB, Belsky J. Epidemiologic studies of coronary heart disease and stroke in Japanese men living in Japan, Hawaii and California: prevalence of coronary and hypertensive heart disease and associated risk factors. *Am J Epidemiol* 1975; **102**: 514–25.

[6] Marmot MG. Alcohol and coronary heart disease. *Int J Epidemiol* 1984; **13**: 160–7.

[7] Beaglehole R, Salmond CE, Hooper A, *et al*. Blood pressure and social interaction in Tokelauan migrants in New Zealand. *J Chronic Dis* 1977; **30**: 803–12.

[8] Bonita R, Beaglehole R. Trends in cerebrovascular disease mortality in New Zealand. *NZ Med J* 1982; **95**: 411–4.

[9] Kushi LH, Lew RA, Stare FJ, *et al*. Diet and 20-year mortality from coronary heart disease: the Ireland–Boston Diet-Heart Study. *N Engl J Med* 1985; **312**: 811–8.

[10] Study Group of the European Atherosclerosis Society. Strategies for the prevention of coronary heart disease: a policy statement of the European Atherosclerosis Society. *Eur Heart J* 1987; **8**: 77–88

[11] Rose G. Strategy of prevention: lessons from cardiovascular disease. *BMJ* 1981; **282**: 1847–1851.

[12] Law MR, Wald NJ, Thompson SG. By how much and how quickly does reduction in serum cholesterol concentration lower risk of ischaemic heart disease? *BMJ* 1994; **308**: 367–72.

[13] Law MR, Wald NJ, Wu T, Hackshaw A, Bailey A. Systematic underestimation of association between serum cholesterol concentration and ischaemic heart disease in observational studies: data from the BUPA study. *BMJ* 1994; **308**: 363–6.

[14] Ramsay LE, Yeo WW, Jackson PR. Dietary reduction of serum cholesterol concentration: time to think again. *BMJ* 1991; **303**: 953–7.

[15] Department of Health. Standing Medical Advisory Committee. *Blood cholesterol testing: the cost-effectiveness of opportunistic cholesterol testing.* London: Department of Health, 1990.

[16] Department of Health. *The health of the nation: key area handbook: coronary heart disease and stroke.* Heywood, Lancs: Department of Health, 1993.

[17] Marmot MG, Poulter NR. Primary prevention of stroke. *Lancet* 1992; **339**: 344–7.

[18] Department of Health and Social Security. *Diet and coronary heart disease: report of the Advisory Panel of the Committee on Medical Aspects of Food Policy (Nutrition) on diet in relation to cardiovascular and cerebrovascular disease.* London: HMSO 1974. (Report on Health and Social Subjects; 7).

[19] Department of Health. *The Health of the nation: a strategy for health in England.* London: HMSO, 1992.

[20] Chen Z, Peto R, Collins R, MacMahon S, Lu J, Li W. Serum cholesterol concentration and coronary heart disease in population with low cholesterol concentrations. *BMJ* 1991; **303**: 276–82.

[21] Office of Population Censuses and Surveys. *Mortality Statistics: area 1990.* London: HMSO, 1982 (Series DH5; no 17).

[22] Office of Population Censuses and Surveys. *Morbidity Statistics from General Practice.* MB5 no 1. London: HMSO.

[23] Department of Health. *Hospital Episode Statistics*: Volume 1 Financial year 1989–90. London: Department of Health, 1993.

[24] World Health Organisation. *World Health Statistics Annual 1989.* Geneva: WHO, 1989.

[25] Office of Population Censuses and Surveys. *Occupational mortality: Decennial supplement 1979–80, 1982–83.* London: HMSO, 1986 (Series DS; no 6).

[26] Balarajan R. Ethnic differences in mortality from Ischaemic Heart Disease and Cerebrovascular Disease in England and Wales. *BMJ* 1991; **302**: 560–4.

[27] White A, Nicolaas G, Foster K, Browne F, Carey S. *Health Survey for England 1991: a survey carried out by the Social Survey Division of the OPCS on behalf of the Department of Health.* London: HMSO, 1993.(Series HS; no 1).

[28] Office of Population Censuses and Surveys. *The heights and weights of adults in Great Britain.* London: HMSO, 1984 (SS 1138).

[29] Allied Dunbar, Sports Council and Health Education Authority. *Allied Dunbar National Fitness Survey.* London: Sports Council/Health Education Authority, 1992.

[30] Office of Population Censuses and Surveys. OPCS Monitor, General Household Survey: Cigarette Smoking 1972 to 1990. Government Statistical Service, 26 November 1991. London: Office of Population Censuses and Surveys, 1991 (Series SS 91/3).

[31] Ministry of Agriculture, Fisheries and Food. *Household food consumption and expenditure 1990, 1991, 1992.* London: HMSO, 1991, 1992, 1993.

[32] Organisation for Economic Co-operation and Development. *Food Consumption Statistics 1979–1988.* Paris: OECD, 1991.

[33] Ministry of Agriculture, Fisheries and Food. *The Dietary and Nutritional Survey of British Adults – Further Analysis*. London: HMSO, 1994.

[34] McGill HC. The lesion. In: Schettler G, Weizel A, eds. *Atherosclerosis III*. Berlin: Springer, 1974: 27–38.

[35] Restrepo C, Tracy RE. Variation in human aortic fatty streaks among geographic locations. *Atherosclerosis* 1975; **21**: 179–93.

[36] Tejada C, Strong JP, Montenegro MR, Restrepo C, Solberg LA. Distribution of coronary and aortic atherosclerosis by geographic location, age and sex. *Lab Invest* 1968; **18**: 509–26.

[37] Strong JP, Solberg LA, Restrepo C. Atherosclerosis in persons with coronary heart disease. *Lab Invest* 1968; **18**: 527–37.

[38] Freedman DS, Newman WP, Tracy RE, *et al*. Black-white differences in aortic fatty streaks in adolescence and early adulthood: the Bogalusa Heart Study. *Circulation* 1988; **77**: 856–64.

[39] Faggiotto A, Ross R. Studies of hypercholesterolemia in the nonhuman primate. II. Fatty streak conversion to fibrous plaque. *Arteriosclerosis* 1984; **4**: 341–56.

[40] Dupree RH, Fields RI, McMahan, CA, Strong JP. Atherosclerotic lesions and coronary heart disease: key relationships in necropsied cases. *Lab Invest* 1973; **28**, 252–62.

[41] PDAY Research group. Relationship of atherosclerosis in young men to serum lipoprotein cholesterol concentrations and smoking: a preliminary report from the Pathobiological Determinants of Atherosclerosis in Youth (PDAY) Research Group. JAMA 1990: **264**: 3018–24.

[42] Steinberg D, Parthasarathy S, Carew TE, Khoo JC, Witztum JL. Beyond cholesterol: modifications of low density lipoprotein that increase its atherogenicity. *N Engl J Med* 1989; **320**: 915–24.

[43] Witztum JL, Steinberg D. Role of oxidised low density lipoprotein in atherogenesis. *J Clin Invest* 1991; **88**: 1785–92.

[44] Berliner JA, Territo M, Sevanian A, *et al*. Minimally modified low density lipoprotein stimulates monocyte endothelial interactions. *J Clin Invest* 1990; **85**: 1260–6.

[45] Goldstein JL, Ho YK, Basu SK, Brown MS. Binding site on macrophages that mediates uptake and degradation of acetylated low density lipoprotein, producing massive cholesterol deposition. *Proc Natl Acad Sci USA* 1979; **76**: 333–7.

[46] Ross R. The pathogenesis of atherosclerosis – an update. *N Engl J Med* 1986; **314**: 488–500.

[47] Lever MJ. Haemodynamic factors. In: Biology and Pathology of the Vessel Wall. N Woolf (ed). New York: Praeger 1983.

[48] Thomas AC, Knapman PA, Krikler DM, Davies MJ. Community study of the causes of "natural" sudden death. *BMJ* 1988; **297**: 1453–6.

[49] Davies MJ, Thomas A. Thrombosis and acute coronary-artery lesions in sudden cardiac ischemic death. *N Engl J Med* 1984; **310**: 1137–40.

[50] Warnes C, Roberts WC. Comparison at necropsy by age group of amount and distribution of narrowing by atherosclerotic plaque in 2995 five-mm long segments of 240 major coronary arteries in 60 men aged 31 to 70 years with sudden coronary death. *Am Heart J* 1984; **108**: 431–5.

[51] Lo YS, Cutler JE, Blake K, Wright AM, Kron J, Swerdlow CD. Angiographic coronary morphology in survivors of cardiac arrest. *Am Heart J* 1988; **115**: 781–5.

[52] Stevenson WG, Wiener I, Yeatman L, Wohlgelernter D, Weiss JN. Complicated atherosclerotic lesions: a potential cause of ischemic ventricular arrhythmias in cardiac arrest survivors who do not have inducible ventricular tachycardia. *Am Heart J* 1988: **116**: 1–6.

[53] Davies MJ. Morphology and natural history of atherosclerotic lesions in the human artery tree. In: Davies MJ, Woolf N, eds. *Atheroma: atherosclerosis in ischaemic heart disease. Vol 1: the mechanisms*. London: Science Press, 1990; 2.1–2.52.

[54] Woolf N. Thrombosis and atherosclerosis. In: Bloom AL, Thomas DP, eds. *Haemostasis and thrombosis*. 2nd ed. Edinburgh: Churchill Livingstone, 1987; 651–78.

[55] Woolf N, Bradley JW, Crawford T, Carstairs KC. Experimental mural thrombosis in the pig aorta: the early natural history. *Br J Exp Pathol* 1968; **49**: 257–64.

[56] Meade TW. Epidemiology of atheroma, thrombosis and ischaemic heart disease. In: Bloom AL, Thomas DP, eds. *Haemostasis and thrombosis*. 2nd ed. Edinburgh: Churchill Livingstone, 1987; 697–720.

[57] Meade TW, Imeson J, Stirling Y. Effects of changes in smoking and other characteristics on clotting factors and the risk of ischaemic heart disease. *Lancet* 1987; **2**: 986–8.

[58] Kannel WB, Wolf PA. In: Russell RWR, ed *Vascular Diseases of the Central Nervous System*, Churchill Livingstone, Edinburgh, 1983; 1.

[59] Law MR, Thompson SG, Wald NJ. Assessing possible hazards of reducing serum cholesterol. *BMJ* 1994; **308**: 373–9.

[60] British Nutrition Foundation. Task Force on Trans Fatty Acids. *Trans fatty acids: report of the British Nutrition Foundation's Task Force*. London: British Nutrition Foundation, 1987.

[61] Brisson GJ. *Lipids in human nutrition: an appraisal of some dietary concepts*. Lancaster: MTP Press, 1982.

[62] Kiritsakis A, Aspris P, Markakis P. Trans isomerisation of certain vegetable oils during frying. *Developments in Food Science* 1990; **24** (Flavors and off-flavors '89): 893–6.

[63] International Association of Fish Meal Manufacturers. *Dietary trans unsaturated fatty acids and cardiovascular disease: a review submitted to the DHSS by the Association of Fish Meal Manufacturers*. Potters Bar: The Association, 1986.

[64] Leake DS. Effects of mildly oxidized low-density lipoprotein on endothelial cell function. *Curr Opin Lipidology* 1991; **2**: 301–5.

[65] Hegsted DM. Serum-cholesterol response to dietary cholesterol: a re-evaluation. *Am J Clin Nutr* 1986; **44**: 299–305.

[66] Goldstein JL, Brown MS. The low density lipoprotein pathway and its relation to atherosclerosis. *Annu Rev Biochem* 1977; **46**: 897–930.

[67] Needleman P, Moncada S, Bunting S, Vane JR, Hamberg M, Samuelsson B. Identification of an enzyme in platelet microsomes which generates thromboxane A2 from prostaglandin endoperoxides. *Nature* 1976; **261**: 558–60.

[68] Bunting S, Moncada S, Vane JR. The effects of prostagladin endoperoxides and thromboxane A2 on strips of rabbit coeliac artery and certain other smooth muscle preparations. *Br J Pharmacol* 1976; **57**: 462P–3P.

[69] Department of Health. *Dietary sugars and human disease: report of the Panel on Dietary Sugars, Committee on Medical Aspects of Food Policy*. London: HMSO, 1989. (Report on Health and Social Subjects; 37).

[70] Alberti KGMM, Hockaday TDR. Diabetes Mellitus. In: Weatherall DJ *et al*, eds. *Oxford Textbook of Medicine (Second Edition)*, Volume 1. Oxford: Oxford University Press, 1987; 9.51–9.101.

[71] British Nutrition Foundation. *Complex carbohydrates in foods: the report of the British Nutrition Foundation's Task Force*. London: Chapman & Hall for the British Nutrition Foundation, 1990.

[72] Martin MJ, Hulley SB, Browner WS, Kuller LH, Wentworth D. Serum cholesterol, blood pressure, and mortality: implications from a cohort of 361,662 men. *Lancet* 1986; **2**: 933–6.

[73] Goldbourt V, Holtzman E, Neufeld HN. Total and high density lipoprotein cholesterol in the serum and risk of mortality: evidence of a threshold effect. *BMJ* 1985; **290**: 1239–43.

[74] Reed D, Yano K, Kagan A. Lipids and lipoproteins as predictors of coronary heart disease, stroke, and cancer in the Honolulu Heart Program. *Am J Med* 1986; **80**: 871–8.

[75] Rose G, Shipley M. Plasma cholesterol concentration and death from coronary heart disease: 10-year results of the Whitehall study. *BMJ* 1986; **293**: 306–7.

[76] Pocock SJ, Shaper AG, Phillips AN. Concentrations of high density lipoprotein cholesterol, triglycerides, and total cholesterol in ischaemic heart disease. *BMJ* 1989; **298**: 998–1002.

[77] Keys A, ed. Coronary heart disease in seven countries. *Circulation* 1970; **41**(4 Suppl): I1–211.

[78] Robertson TL, Kato H, Gordon T, *et al*. Epidemiologic studies of coronary heart disease and stroke in Japanese men living in Japan, Hawaii and California: coronary heart disease risk factors in Japan and Hawaii. *Am J Cardiol* 1977; **39**: 244–9.

[79] Chen J, Campbell TC, Li J, Peto R. *Diet, life-style and mortality in China: a study of the characteristics of 65 Chinese counties*. Oxford: OUP, 1990.

[80] Hatano S. Changing CHD mortality and its causes in Japan during 1955–1985. *Int J Epidemiol* 1989, **18** (3 Suppl 1): S149–58.

[81] Slack J. Risks of ischaemic heart-disease in familial hyperlipoproteinaemic states. *Lancet* 1969; **2**: 1380–2.

[82] Stone NJ, Levy RI, Fredrickson DS, Verter J. Coronary artery disease in 116 kindred with familial type II hyperlipoproteinemia. *Circulation* 1974; **49**: 476–88.

[83] Fuller WA. *Measurement error models*. New York: Wiley, 1987.

[84] Yusuf S, Wittes J, Freidman L. Overview of results of randomized clinical trials in heart disease: II. Unstable angina, heart failure, primary prevention with aspirin, and risk factor modification. *JAMA* 1988; **260**: 2259–63.

[85] Holme I. An analysis of randomized trials evaluating the effect of cholesterol reduction on total mortality and coronary heart disease incidence. *Circulation* 1990; **82**: 1916–24.

[86] National Academy of Sciences. Committee on Diet and Health. *Diet and health: implications for reducing chronic disease risk.* Washington DC: National Academy Press, 1989.

[87] Miller GJ, Miller NE. Plasma-high-density-lipoprotein concentration and development of ischaemic heart disease. *Lancet* 1975; **1**: 16–9.

[88] Cohn K, Sakai FJ, Langston MF. Effect of clofibrate on progression of coronary disease: a prospective angiographic study in man. *Am Heart J* 1975; **89**: 591–8.

[89] Knight L, Scheibel R, Amplatz K, Varco RL, Buchwald H. Radiographic appraisal of the Minnesota partial ileal bypass study. *Surg Forum* 1972; **23**: 141–2.

[90] Brensike JF, Levy RI, Kelsey SF *et al*. Effects of therapy with cholestyramine on progression of coronary arteriosclerosis: results of the NHLBI Type II Coronary Intervention Study. *Circulation* 1984; **69**: 313–24.

[91] Blankenhorn DH, Nessim SA, Johnson RL, Sanmarco ME, Azen SP, Cashin-Hemphill L. Beneficial effects of combined colestipol-niacin therapy on coronary atherosclerosis and coronary venous bypass grafts. *JAMA* 1987; **257**: 3233–40.

[92] Brown G, Albers JJ, Fisher LD, et al. Regression of coronary artery disease as a result of intensive lipid-lowering therapy in men with high levels of apolipoprotein B. *N Engl J Med* 1990; 323: 1289-98.

[93] Watts GF, Lewis B, Brunt JNH, Lewis ES, Coltart DJ, Smith LDR, Mann JI, Swan AV. Effects on coronary artery disease of lipid-lowering diet, or diet plus cholestyramine, in the St Thomas' Atherosclerosis Regression Study (STARS). *Lancet* 1992; **339**: 563–69.

[94] Buchwald H, Varco RL, Matts JP, *et al*. Effect of partial ileal bypass surgery on mortality and morbidity from coronary heart disease in patients with hypercholesterolemia: report of the Program on the Surgical Control of the Hyperlipidemias (POSCH). *N Engl J Med* 1990; **323**: 946–55.

[95] Jacobs D, Blackburn H, Higgins M, Reed D, Iso H *et al*. Report of the Conference on Low Cholesterol:Mortality Associations. *Circulation* 1992; **86**: 1046–60.

[96] Rose G, Blackburn H, Keys A, *et al*. Colon cancer and blood-cholesterol. *Lancet* 1974; **1**: 181–3.

[97] Rose G, Shipley M. Plasma lipids and mortality: a source of error. *Lancet* 1980; **1**: 523–6.

[98] Klag MJ, Ford DE, Mead LA, *et al*. Serum cholesterol in young men and subsequent cardiovascular disease. *N Engl J Med* 1993; **328**: 313–8.

[99] Marmot M. The cholesterol papers: lowering population cholesterol concentrations probably isn't harmful. *BMJ* 1994; **308**: 351–2.

[100] Vitols S, Gahrton G, Bjorkholm M, Peterson C. Hypocholesterolaemia in malignancy due to elevated low-density-lipoprotein-receptor activity in tumour cells: evidence from studies in patients with leukaemia. *Lancet* 1985; **2**: 1150–4.

[101] Budd D, Ginsberg H. Hypocholesterolemia and acute myelogenous leukemia: association between disease activity and plasma low-density lipoprotein cholesterol concentrations. *Cancer* 1986; **58**: 1361–5.

[102]. Davey-Smith G, Pekkanen J. Should there be a moratorium on the use of cholesterol lowering drugs? *BMJ* 1992; **304**: 431–4.

[103] Winawer SJ, Flehinger BJ, Buchalter J, Herbert E, Shike M. Declining serum cholesterol levels prior to diagnosis of colon cancer: a time-trend, case-control study. *JAMA* 1990; **263**: 2083–5.

[104] Kozarevic D, McGee D, Vojvodic N, *et al.* Serum cholesterol and mortality: the Yugoslavia cardiovascular disease study. *Am J Epidemiol* 1981; **114**: 21–8.

[105] Isles CG, Hole DJ, Gillis CR, Hawthorne VM, Lever AF. Plasma cholesterol, coronary heart disease, and cancer in the Renfrew and Paisley survey. *Br Med J* 1989; **298**: 920–4.

[106] Muldoon MF, Manuck SB, Matthews KA. Lowering cholesterol concentrations and mortality: a quantitative review of primary prevention trials. *BMJ* 1990; **301**: 309–14.

[107] Ravnskov U. Cholesterol lowering trials in coronary heart disease: frequency of citation and outcome. *BMJ* 1992; **305**: 15–9.

[108] Davey-Smith G, Song F, Sheldon TA. Cholesterol lowering and mortality: the importance of considering initial level of risk. *BMJ* 1993; **306**: 1367–73.

[109] Rhoads GG, Dahlen G, Berg K, Morton NE, Daneberg AL. Lp(a) lipoprotein as a risk factor for myocardial infarction. *JAMA* 1986; **256**: 2540–4.

[110] Seed M, Hoppichler F, Reaveley D, *et al.* Relation of serum lipoprotein(a) concentration and apolipoprotein(a) phenotype to coronary heart disease in patients with familial hypercholesterolaemia. *New Eng J Med* 1990; **322**: 1494–9.

[111] Sandkamp M, Funke H, Schulte H, Kohler E, Assmann G. Lipoprotein(a) is an independent risk factor for myocardial infarction at a young age. *Clin Chem* 1990; **36**: 20–3.

[112] Jauhiainen M, Koskinen P, Ehnholm C, *et al.* Lipoprotein (a) and coronary heart disease risk: a nested case-control study of the Helsinki Heart Study participants. *Atherosclerosis* 1991; **89**: 59–67.

[113] Ridker PM, Hennekens CH, Stampfer MJ. A prospective study of lipoprotein (a) and the risk of myocardial infarction. *JAMA* 1993; **270**: 2195–9.

[114] Haberland ME, Fless GM, Scanu AM, Fogelman AM. Modification of Lp(a) by malondialdehyde leads to rapid uptake by human monocytes-macrophages. *Arterisclerosis* 1989; **9**: 700 (abstract).

[115] Loscalzo J, Weinfeld M, Fless G, Scanu AM. Lipoprotein(a), fibrin binding and plasminogen activation. *Arteriosclerosis* 1990; **10**: 240–5.

[116] Stamler J, Neaton JD, Wentworth DN. Blood pressure (systolic and diastolic) and risk of fatal coronary heart disease. *Hypertension* 1989; **13** (5 Suppl): I2–I12.

[117] MacMahon S, Peto R, Cutler J, *et al.* Blood pressure, stroke, and coronary heart disease. Part 1, prolonged differences in blood pressure: prospective observational studies corrected for the regression dilution bias. *Lancet* 1990; **335**: 765–74.

[118] Chobanian AV, Brecher PI, Haudenschild CC. Effects of hypertension and of antihypertensive therapy on atherosclerosis. *Hypertension* 1986; **8**(4 Suppl I): I15–21.

[119] Collins R, Peto R, MacMahon S, *et al.* Blood pressure, stroke, and coronary heart disease. Part 2, short-term reductions in blood pressure: overview of randomised drug trials in their epidemiological context. *Lancet* 1990; **335**: 827–38.

[120] World Health Organisation. Study group on diet, nutrition and prevention on noncommunicable diseases. *Diet, nutrition and the prevention of chronic diseases: report of a WHO study group*. Geneva: WHO, 1990. (Technical Report Series; 797).

[121] Hubert HB, Feinleib M, McNamara PM, Castelli WP. Obesity as an independent risk factor for cardiovascular disease: a 26-year follow-up of participants in the Framingham Heart Study. *Circulation* 1983; **67**: 968–77.

[122] Rabkin SW, Mathewson FA, Hsu PH. Relation of body weight to development of ischemic heart disease in a cohort of young North American men after a 26-year observation period: the Manitoba Study. *Am J Cardiol* 1977; **39**: 452–8.

[123] Jarrett RJ, Shipley MJ, Rose G. Weight and mortality in the Whitehall Study. *BMJ* 1982; **285**: 535–7.

[124] Imeson JD, Haines AP, Meade TW. Skinfold thickness, body mass index and ischaemic heart disease. *J Epidemiol Community Health* 1989; **43**: 223–7.

[125] Ducimetiere P, Richard J, Cambien F. The pattern of subcutaneous fat distribution in middle-aged men and the risk of coronary heart disease: the Paris Prospective Study. *Int J Obes* 1986; **10**: 229–40.

[126] Lapidus L, Bengtsson C, Larsson B, Pennert K, Rybo E, Sjostrom L. Distribution of adipose tissue and risk of cardiovascular disease and death: a 12-year follow-up of participants in the population study of women in Gothenburg, Sweden. *BMJ* 1984; **289**: 1257–61.

[127] Larsson B, Svardsudd K, Welin L, Wilhelmsen L, Bjorntorp P, Tibblin G. Abdominal adipose tissue distribution, obesity, and risk of cardiovascular disease and death: 13-year follow-up of participants in the study of men born in 1913. *BMJ* 1984; **288**: 1401–4.

[128] Noppa H. Body weight change in relation to incidence of ischemic heart disease and change in risk factors for ischemic heart disease. *Am J Epidemiol* 1980; **111**: 693–704.

[129] Hubert HB, Eaker ED, Garrison RJ, Castelli WP. Life-style correlates of risk factor change in young adults: an eight-year study of coronary heart disease risk factors in the Framingham offspring. *Am J Epidemiol* 1987; **125**: 812–31.

[130] Olefsky JM, Reaven GM, Farquhar JW. Effects of weight reduction on obesity: studies of lipid and carbohydrate and metabolism in normal and hyperlipoprotinemic subjects. *J Clin Invest* 1974; **53**: 64–76.

[131] Hamm P, Shekelle RB, Stamler J. Large fluctuations in body weight during young adulthood and twenty-five year risk of coronary death in men. *Am J Epidemiol* 1989; **129**: 312–8.

[132] Lissner L, Odell PM, D'Agostino RB, *et al*. Variability of body weight and health outcomes in the Framingham population. *N Engl J Med* 1991; **324**: 1839–44.

[133] Jeffery RW, Wing RR, French SA. Weight cycling and cardiovascular risk factors in obese men and women. *Am J Clin Nutr* 1992; **55**: 641–4.

[134] Modan M, Halkin H, Almog S, *et al*. Hyperinsulinemia – a link between hypertension, obesity and glucose intolerance. *J Clin Invest* 1985; **75**: 809–17.

[135] Reaven GM. Role of insulin resistance in human disease. *Diabetes* 1988; **37**: 1595–607.

[136] McKeigue PM, Shah B, Marmot MG. Relation of central obesity and insulin resistance with high diabetes prevalence and cardiovascular risk in South Asians. *Lancet* 1991; **337**: 382–6.

[137] Garrow JS. Importance of obesity. *BMJ* 1991; **303**: 704–6.

[138] Barker DJ, Winter PD, Osmond C, Margetts B, Simmonds SJ. Weight in infancy and death from ischaemic heart disease. *Lancet* 1989; **ii**: 577–80.

[139] Barker DJ, Bull AR, Osmond C, Simmonds SJ. Fetal and placental size and risk of hypertension in adult life. *BMJ* 1990; **301**: 259–62.

[140] Barker DJ, Meade TW, Fall CH, Lee A, Osmond C, Phipps K, Stirling Y. Relation of fetal and infant growth to plasma fibrinogen and factor VII concentrations in adult life. *BMJ* 1992; **304**: 148–52.

[141] Barker DJ, Martyn CN, Osmond C, Hales CN, Fall CHD. Growth in utero and serum cholesterol concentrations in adult life. *Br Med J* 1993; **307**: 1524–7.

[142] Hales CN, Barker DJ, Clark PM, *et al*. Fetal and infant growth and impaired glucose tolerance at age 64. *BMJ* 1991; **303**: 1019–22.

[143] Osmond C, Barker DPJ, Winter PD, Fall CHD, Simmonds SJ. Early growth and death from cardiovascular disease in women. *Br Med J* 1993; **307**: 1519–24.

[144] Fall CH, Barker DJ, Osmond C, Winter PD, Clark PM, Hales CN. Relation of infant feeding to adult serum cholesterol concentration and death from ischaemic heart disease. BMJ 1992; 304: 801–5.

[145] Fuller JH, Shipley MJ, Rose G, Jarrett RJ, Keen H. Mortality from coronary heart disease and stroke in relation to degree of glycaemia: the Whitehall study. *BMJ* 1983; **287**: 867–70.

[146] Marshall JA, Hamman RF, Baxter J. High-fat, low-carbohydrate diet and the etiology of non-insulin-dependent diabetes mellitus: the San Luis Valley Diabetes Study. *Am J Epidemiol* 1991; **134**: 590–603.

[147] Pyorala K, Savolainen E, Kaukola S, Haapakoski J. Plasma insulin as coronary heart disease risk factor: relationship to other risk factors and predictive value during 9½-year follow-up of the Helsinki Policemen Study population. *Acta Med Scand* 1985; (Suppl 701): 38–52.

[148] Welborn TA, Wearne K. Coronary heart disease incidence and cardiovascular mortality in Busselton with reference to glucose and insulin concentrations. *Diabetes Care* 1979; **2**: 154–60.

[149] Eschwege E, Richard JL, Thibult N *et al*. Coronary heart disease mortality in relation with diabetes, blood glucose and plasma insulin levels: the Paris Prospective Study, ten years later. *Horm Metab Res* 1985; (Suppl 15): 41–46.

[150] Fontbonne A *et al*. Hyperinsulinaemia as a predictor of coronary disease mortality in a healthy population: the Paris prospective study, 15-year follow up. *Diabetologia* 1991; **34**: 356–61.

[151] Haffner SM, Valdez RA, Hazuda HP, Mitchell BD, Morales PA, Stern MP. Prospective analysis of the Insulin-Resistance Syndrome (Syndrome X). *Diabetes* 1992; **41**: 715–22.

[152] McKeigue PM, Miller GJ, Marmot MG. Coronary heart disease in South Asians overseas: a review. *J Clin Epidemiol* 1989; **42**: 597–609.

[153] Parker DR, Weiss ST, Troisi R, Cassano PA, Vokonas PS, Landsberg L. Relationship of dietary saturated fatty acids and body habitus to serum insulin concentrations: the Normative Aging Study. *Am J Clin Nutr* 1993; **58**: 129–36.

[154] Maron DJ, Fair JM, Haskell WL. Saturated fat intake and insulin resistance in men with coronary artery disease. *Circulation* 1991; **84**: 2020–7.

[155] Meade TW, Mellows S, Brozovic M, *et al*. Haemostatic function and ischaemic heart disease: principal results of the Northwick Park Heart Study. *Lancet* 1986; **2**: 533–7.

[156] Ranby M. Studies on the kinetics of plasminogen activation by tissue plasminogen activator. *Biochim Biophys Acta* 1982; **704**: 461–9.

[157] Fuchs HE, Berger H, Pizzo SV. Catabolism of human tissue plasminogen activator. *Blood* 1985; **65**: 539–44.

[158] Lambers JW, Cammenga M, Konig BW, Mertens K, Pannekoek H, van Mourick JA. Activation of human endothelial cell-type plasminogen activator inhibitor (PAI-1) by negatively charged phospholipids. *J Biol Chem* 1987; **262**: 17492–6.

[159] Hamsten A, de Faire U, Walldius G, *et al*. Plasminogen activator inhibitor in plasma: risk factor for recurrent myocardial infarction. *Lancet* 1987; **2**: 3–10.

[160] Berdeaux DH, Marlar RA. Report of an American family with elevated plasminogen activator inhibitor as a cause of multiple thromboses: response to prednisone. *Thromb Haemost* 1991; **65**: 1044 (abstract 1254).

[161] Meade TW, Ruddock V, Stirling Y, Chakrabarti R, Miller GJ. Fibrinolytic activity, clotting factors, and the long term incidence of ischaemic heart disease in the Northwick Park Heart Study. *Lancet* 1993; **342**: 1076–9.

[162] Doll R, Peto R. Mortality in relation to smoking: 20 years' observations on male British doctors. *BMJ* 1976; **2**: 1525–36.

[163] Mann JI, Doll R, Thorogood M, Vessey MP, Waters WE. Risk factors for myocardial infarction in young women. *Br J Prev Soc Med* 1976; **30**: 94–100.

[164] Pooling Project Research Group. Relationship of blood pressure, serum cholesterol, smoking habit, relative weight and ECG abnormalities to incidence of major coronary events: final report of the Pooling Project. *J Chronic Dis* 1978; **31**: 201–306.

[165] Reid DD, Hamilton PJ, McCartney P, Rose G, Jarrett RJ, Keen H. Smoking and other risk factors for coronary heart-disease in British civil servants. *Lancet* 1976; **2**: 979–84.

[166] Bonita R, Scragg R, Stewart A, Jackson R, Beaglehole R. Cigarette smoking and risk of premature stroke in men and women. *BMJ* 1986; **293**: 6–8.

[167] Bell BA, Symon L. Smoking and subarachnoid haemorrhage. *BMJ* 1979; **1**: 577–8.

[168] Kannel WB, McGee DL. Update on some epidemiologic features of intermittent claudication: the Framingham Study. *J Am Geriatr Soc* 1985; **33**: 13–8.

[169] Craig WY, Palomaki GE, Haddow JE. Cigarette smoking and serum lipid and lipoprotein concentrations: an analysis of published data. *BMJ* 1989; **298**: 784–8.

[170] Wilhelmsen L, Svardsudd K, Korsan-Bengtsen K, Larsson B, Welin L, Tibblin G. Fibrinogen as a risk factor for stroke and myocardial infarction. *N Engl J Med* 1984; **311**: 501–5.

[171] Stone MC, Thorp JM. Plasma fibrinogen – a major coronary risk factor. In: Lenzi S, Descovich GC, eds. *Atherosclerosis and cardiovascular diseases*. Bologna: Editrice Compositori, 1984; 3–10.

[172] Kannel WB, Wolf PA, Castelli WP, D'Agostino RB. Fibrinogen and risk of cardiovascular disease: the Framingham study. *JAMA* 1987; **258**: 1183–6.

[173] Fehily AM, Phillips KM, Yarnell JW. Diet, smoking, social class, and body mass index in the Caerphilly Heart Disease Study. *Am J Clin Nutr* 1984; **40**: 827–33.

[174] Bolton-Smith C, Casey CE, Gey KF, Smith WCS, Tunstall-Pedoe H. Antioxidant vitamin intakes assessed using a foo-frequency questionnaire: correlation with biochemical status in smokers and non-smokers. *Br J Nutr* 1991; **65**: 337–46.

[175] Schectman G, Byrd JC, Hoffmann R. Ascorbic acid requirements for smokers: analysis of a population survey. *Am J Clin Nutr* 1991; **53**: 1466–70.

[176] Kallner A, Hartmann D, Hornig D. On the requirements of ascorbic acid in man: steady-state turnover and body pool in smokers. *Am J Clin Nutr* 1981; **34**: 1347–55.

[177] Harats D, Ben-Naim M, Dabach Y, Hollander G, Stein O, Stein Y. Cigarette smoking renders LDL susceptible to peroxidative modification and enhanced metabolism by macrophages. *Atherosclerosis* 1989; **79**: 245–52.

[178] Duthie GG, Wahle KWJ, James WPT. Oxidants, antioxidants and cardiovascular disease. *Nutr Res Rev* 1989; **2**: 51–62.

[179] Lund-Larsen PG, Tretli S. Changes in smoking habits and body weight after a three year period – the cardiovascular disease study in Finnmark. *J Chronic Dis* 1982; **35**: 773–80.

[180] Gordon T, Kannel WB, Dawber TR, McGee D. Changes associated with quitting cigarette smoking: the Framingham Study. *Am Heart J* 1975; **90**: 322–8.

[181] Friedman GD, Siegelaub AB. Changes after quitting cigarette smoking. *Circulation* 1980; **61**: 716–23.

[182] Stubbe I, Eskilsson J, Nilsson-Ehle P. High-density lipoprotein concentrations increase after stopping smoking. *BMJ* 1982; **284**: 1511–3.

[183] Tuomilehto J, Tanskanen A, Salonen JT, Nissinen A, Koskela K. Effects of smoking and stopping smoking on serum high-density lipoprotein cholesterol levels in a representative population sample. *Prev Med* 1986; **15**: 35–45.

[184] Shapiro S, Slone D, Rosenberg L, Kaufman DW, Stolley PD, Miettinen OS. Oral-contraceptive use in relation to myocardial infarction. *Lancet* 1979; **1**: 743–7.

[185] Ballor DL, Keesey RE. A meta-analysis of the factors affecting exercise-induced changes in body mass, fat mass and fat-free mass in males and females. *Int J Obes* 1991; **15**: 717–26.

[186] Wood PD, Terry RB, Haskell WL. Metabolism of substrates; diet, lipoprotein metabolism and exercise. *Fed Proc* 1985; **44**: 358–63.

[187] Wood PD, Stefanick ML, Williams PT, Haskell WL. The effects on plasma lipoproteins of a prudent weight-reducing diet, with or without exercise, in overweight men and women. *N Engl J Med* 1991; **325**: 461–6.

[188] Powell KE, Thompson PD, Caspersen CJ, Kendrick JS. Physical activity and the incidence of coronary heart disease. *Annu Rev Public Health* 1987; **8**: 253–87.

[189] Morris JN, Everitt MG, Pollard R, Chave SPW. Vigorous exercise in leisure-time: protection against coronary heart disease. *Lancet* 1980; **2**: 1207–10.

[190] Morris JN, Clayton DG, Everitt MG, Semmence AM, Burgess EH. Exercise in leisure time: coronary attack and death rates. *Br Heart J* 1990; **63**: 325–34.

[191] Paffenbarger RS, Hyde RT, Wing AL, Hsieh C-C. Physical activity, all-cause mortality, and longevity of college alumni. *N Engl J Med* 1986; **314**: 605–13.

[192] Shaper AG, Wannamethee G. Physical activity and ischaemic heart disease in middle-aged British men. *Br Heart J* 1991; **66**: 384–94.

[193] Andrew M, Carter C, O'Brodovich H, Heigenhauser G. Increases in factor VIII complex and fibrolytic activity are dependent on exercise intensity. *J Appl Physiol* 1986; **60**: 1917–22.

[194] Hardman AE, Hudson A, Jones PR, Norgan NG. Brisk walking and plasma high density lipoprotein cholesterol in previously sedentary women. *BMJ* 1989; **299**: 1204–5.

[195] Wood PD, Haskell WL, Blair SN, et al. Increased exercise level and plasma lipoprotein concentrations: a one-year, randomized, controlled study in sedentary, middle-aged men. *Metabolism* 1983; **32**: 31–9.

[196] Nelson L, Jennings GL, Esler MD and Korner PI. Effect of changing levels of physical activity on blood-pressure and haemodynamics in essential hypertension. *Lancet* 1986; **ii**: 473–6.

[197] Hagberg JM, Montain SJ, Martin WH, Ehsani AA. Effect of exercise training in 60- to 69-year-old persons with essential hypertension. *Am J Cardiol* 1989; **64**: 348–53.

[198] Martin JE, Dubbert PM, Cushman WC. Controlled trial of aerobic exercise in hypertension. *Circulation* 1990; **81**: 1560–7.

[199] Somers VK, Conway J, Johnston J, Sleight P. Effects of endurance training on baroreflex sensitivity and blood pressure in borderline hypertension. *Lancet* 1991; **337**: 1363–8.

[200] Roman O, Camuzzi AL, Villalon E, Klenner C. Physical training programme in arterial hypertension: a long-term prospective follow-up. *Cardiology* 1981; **67**: 230–43.

[201] Horton ES. Exercise and physical training: effects on insulin sensitivity and glucose metabolism. D*iabetes Metab Rev* 1986; **2**: 1–17.

[202] Bjorntorp P, Fahlen M, Grimby G, *et al.* Carbohydrate and lipid metabolism in middle-aged, physically well-trained men. *Metabolism* 1972; **21**: 1037–44.

[203] Helmrich SP, Ragland DR, Leung RW, Paffenbarger RS. Physical activity and reduced occurrence of non-insulin-dependent diabetes mellitus. *N Engl J Med* 1991; **325**: 147–52.

[204] Manson JE, Rimm EB, Stampfer MJ, *et al.* Physical activity and incidence of non-insulin-dependent diabetes mellitus in women. *Lancet* 1991; **338**: 774–8.

[205] Paffenbarger RS, Wing AL, Hyde RT. Physical activity as an index of heart attack risk in college alumni. *Am J Epidemiol* 1978; **108**: 161–75.

[206] Connelly JB, Cooper JA, Meade TW. Strenuous exercise, plasma fibrinogen, and factor VII activity. *Br Heart J* 1992; **67**: 351–4.

[207] Bourey RE, Santoro SA. Interactions of exercise, coagulation, platelets, and fibrinolysis – a brief review. *Med Sci Sports Exerc* 1988; **20**: 439–46.

[208] Watts EJ, Weir P. Reduced platelet aggregation in long-distance runners. *Lancet* 1989; **i**: 1013.

[209] Keys A, Anderson JT, Grande F. Prediction of serum-cholesterol responses of man to changes in fats in the diet. *Lancet* 1957; **ii**: 959–66.

[210] Keys A, Anderson JT, Grande F. Serum cholesterol response to changes in the diet. *Metabolism* 1965; **14**: 747–87.

[211] Hegsted DM, McGandy RB, Myers ML, Stare FJ. Quantitative effects of dietary fat on serum cholesterol in man. *Am J Clin Nutr* 1965; **17**: 281–95.

[212] Brown MS, Goldstein JL. A receptor-mediated pathway for cholesterol homeostasis. *Science* 1986; **232**: 34–47.

[213] Mensink RP. Effects of the individual saturated fatty acids on serum lipids and lipoprotein concentrations. *Am J Clin Nutr* 1993; **57(S)**: 711S–4S.

[214] Bonanome A, Grundy SM. Effect of dietary stearic acid on plasma cholesterol and lipoprotein levels. *N Engl J Med* 1988; **318:** 1244–48.

[215] Hegsted DM, Ansman LM, Johnson JA, Dallal GE. Dietary fat and serum lipids: an evaluation of the experimental data. *Am J Clin Nutr* 1993; **57**: 875–83.

[216] Hayes KC, Khosla P. Dietary fatty acid thresholds and cholesterolemia. *FASEB J* 1992; **6**: 2600–7.

[217] Khosla P, Hayes KC. Comparison between the effects of dietary saturated (16:0), monounsaturated (18:1) and polyunsaturated (18:2) fatty acids on plasma lipoprotein metabolism in cebus and rhesus monkeys fed cholesterol-free diets. *Am J Clin Nutr* 1992; **55**: 51–62.

[218] Mattson FH, Grundy SM. Comparisons of effects of dietary saturated, monounsaturated and polyunsaturated fatty acids on plasma lipids and lipoproteins in man. *J Lipid Res* 1985; **26**: 194–202.

[219] Grundy SM, Nix D, Whelan MF, Franklin L. Comparison of three cholesterol-lowering diets in normolipidemic men. *JAMA* 1986; **256**: 2351–5.

[220] Mensink RP, Katan MB. Effect of monounsaturated fatty acids versus complex carbohydrates on high density lipoproteins in healthy men and women. Lancet 1987; **i**: 122–5.

[221] Baggio G, Pagnan A, Muraca M, *et al.* Olive-oil-enriched diet: effect on serum lipoprotein levels and biliary cholesterol saturation. *Am J Clin Nutr* 1988; **47**: 960–4.

[222] Mensink RP, Katan MB. Effect of a diet enriched with monounsaturated or polyunsaturated fatty acids on levels of low-density and high-density lipoprotein cholesterol in healthy men and women. *N Engl J Med* 1989; **321**: 436–41.

[223] Grundy SM. Monounsaturated fatty acids and cholesterol metabolism: implications for dietary recommendations. *J Nutr* 1989; **119**: 529–33.

[224] Dreon DM, Vranizan KM, Krauss RM, Austin MA, Wood PD. The effects of polyunsaturated fat *vs.* monounsaturated fat on plasma lipoproteins. *JAMA* 1990; **263**: 2462–6.

[225] Berry EM, Eisenberg S, Haratz D, Friedlander Y, Norman Y, Kaufman NA, Stein Y. Effects of diets rich in monounsaturated fatty acids on plasma lipoproteins – the Jerusalem Nutrition Study: High MUFSs *vs* high PUFAs. *Am J Clin Nutr* 1991; **53**: 899–907.

[226] Reaven P, Parthasarathy S, Grasse BJ, *et al.* Feasibility of using an oleate-rich diet to reduce the susceptibility of low-density lipoprotein to oxidative modification in humans. *Am J Clin Nutr* 1991; **54**: 701–6.

[227] Abbey M, Belling GB, Noakes M, Hirata F, Nestel PJ. Oxidation of low density lipoproteins: intra-individual variability and the effect of linoleate supplementation. *Am J Clin Nutr* 1993; **57**: 391–8.

[228] Hodgson JM, Wahlqvist ML, Boxall JA, Balazs ND. Can linoleic acid contribute to coronary artery disease? *Am J Clin Nutr* 1993; **58**: 228–34.

[229] Wood DA, Butler S, Riemersma RA, *et al.* Adipose tissue and platelet fatty acids and coronary heart diseases in Scottish men. *Lancet* 1984; **2**: 117–21.

[230] Wood DA, Riemersma RA, Butler S, *et al.* Linoleic and eicosapentaenoic acids in adipose tissue and platelets and risk of coronary heart disease. *Lancet* 1987; **1**: 177–83.

[231] Blankenhorn DH, Johnson RL, Mack WJ, El Zein HA, Vailas LI. The influence of diet on the appearance of new lesions in human coronary arteries. *JAMA* 1990; **263**: 1646–52.

[232] Sturdevant RA, Pearce ML, Dayton S. Increased prevalence of cholelithiasis in men ingesting a serum-cholesterol-lowering diet. *N Engl J Med* 1973; **288**: 24–7.

[233] National Research Council. Committee on Diet, Nutrition and Cancer. *Diet, nutrition and cancer.* Washington DC: National Academy Press, 1982.

[234] Federation of American Societies for Experimental Biology. Life Sciences Research Office. *Health aspects of dietary 'trans' fatty acids.* Bethesda MD: Federation of American Societies for Experimental Biology, 1985. Report No.: FDA/CFSAN–86/1.

[235] Mensink RP, Katan MB. Effect of dietary trans fatty acids on high-density and low-density lipoprotein cholesterol levels in healthy subjects. *N Engl J Med* 1990; **323**: 439–45.

[236] Zock PL, Katan MB. Hydrogenation alternatives: effects of trans fatty acids and stearic acid versus linoleic acid on serum lipids and lipoproteins in humans. *J Lipid Res* 1992; **33**: 399–410.

[237] Nestel P, Noakes M, Belling B, *et al.* Plasma lipoprotein lipid and Lp(a) changes with substitution of elaidic acid for oleic acid in the diet. *J Lipid Res* 1992; **33**: 1029–36.

[238] Judd JT, Clevidence BA, Muesing RA, Wittes J, Sunkin ME, Podczasy JJ. Dietary trans fatty acids: effects on plasma lipids and lipoproteins of healthy men and women. *Am J Clin Nutr* 1994; **59**: 861–868.

[239] Troisi R, Willett WC, Weiss ST. Trans-fatty acid intake in relation to serum lipid concentrations in adult men. *Am J Clin Nutr* 1992; **56**: 1019–24.

[240] Willett WC, Stampfer MJ, Manson JE, *et al.* Intake of trans fatty acids and risk of coronary heart disease among women. *Lancet* 1993; **341**: 581–5.

[241] Ascherio A, Hennekens CH, Buring JE, Master C, Stampfer MJ, Willett WC. Trans fatty acids intake and risk of myocardial infarction. *Circulation* 1994; **89**: 94–101.

[242] Mensink RP, Zock PL, Katan MB, Hornstra G. Effect of dietary cis and trans fatty acids on serum lipoprotein (a) levels in humans. *J Lipid Res* 1992; **33**: 1493–501.

[243] Hornstra G, van Houwelingen AC, Kester AD, Sundram K. A palm-oil enriched diet lowers serum lipoprotein(a) in normocholesterolemic volunteers. *Atherosclerosis* 1991; **90**: 91–3.

[244] Lichtenstein AH, Ausman LM, Carrasco W, Jenner JL, Ordovas JM, Schaefer EJ. Hydrogenation impairs the hypolipidemic effect of corn oil in humans: hydrogenation, trans fatty acids, and plasma lipids. *Arterioscler Thromb* 1993; **13**: 154–61.

[245] Wahle KWJ, James WPT. Isomeric fatty acids and human health. *Eur J Clin Nutr* 1993; **47**: 828–39.

[246] Edington JD, Geekie M, Carter R, Benfield L, Ball M, Mann J. Serum lipid response to dietary cholesterol in subjects fed a low-fat, high-fiber diet. *Am J Clin Nutr* 1989; **50**: 58–62.

[247] Shekelle RB, Stamler J. Dietary cholesterol and ischaemic heart disease. *Lancet* 1989; **1**: 1177–9.

[248] Dyerberg J, Bang HO. Haemostatic funtion and platelet polyunsaturated fatty acids in Eskimos. *Lancet* 1979; **ii**: 433–5.

[249] Hirai A, Terano T, Hamazaki T, Sajiki J, Kondo S, Ozawa A, Fugita T, Miyamoto T, Tamura Y, Kumagai. The effects of the oral administration of fish oil concentrate on the release and metabolism of [14C] arachidonic acid and [14C] eicosapentanenoic acid by human platelets. *Thromb Res* 1982; **28**: 285–98.

[250] Kromhout D, Bosschieter EB, de Lezenne Coulander C. The inverse relation between fish consumption and 20-year mortality from coronary heart disease. *N Engl J Med* 1985; **312**: 1205–9.

[251] Shekelle RB, Missell L, Paul O, *et al*. Fish consumption and mortality from coronary heart disease. *N Engl J Med* 1985; **313**: 820.

[252] Burr ML, Fehily AM, Gilbert JF, *et al*. Effects of changes in fat, fish and fibre intakes on death and myocardial reinfarction: Diet and Reinfarction Trial (DART). *Lancet* 1989; **ii**: 757–61.

[253] Needleman P, Raz A, Minkes MS, Ferrendelli JA, Sprecher H. Triene prostagladins: prostacylin and thromboxane biosynthesis and unique biological properties. *Proc Natl Acad Sci USA* 1979; **76**: 944–8.

[254] Moncada S, Gryglewski R, Bunting S, Vane JR. An enzyme isolated from arteries transforms prostaglandin endoperoxides to an unstable substance that inhibits platelet aggregation. *Nature* 1976; **263**: 663–5.

[255] Meade TW, Vickers MV, Thompson SG, Stirling Y, Haines AP, Miller GJ. Epidemiological characteristics of platelet aggregability. *BMJ* 1985; **290**: 428–32.

[256] Elwood PC, Renaud S, Sharp DS, Beswick AD, O'Brien JR, Yarnell JW. Ischemic heart disease and platelet aggregation: the Caerphilly Collaborative Heart Disease Study. *Circulation* 1991; **83**: 38–44.

[257] Thorngren M, Gustafson A. Effects of 11-week increases in dietary eicosapentaenoic acid on bleeding time, lipids and platelet aggregation. *Lancet* 1981; **2**: 1190–3.

[258] von Schacky C, Fischer S, Weber PC. Long-term effects of dietary marine omega-3 fatty acids upon plasma and cellular lipids, platelet function, and eicosanoid formation in humans. *J Clin Invest* 1985; **76**: 1626–31.

[259] Pace-Asciak C, Wolfe LS. A novel prostaglandin derivative formed from arachidonic acid by rat stomach homogenates. *Biochemistry* 1971; **10**: 3657–64.

[260] Levenson DJ, Simmons CE, Brenner BM. Arachidonic acid mechanism, prostaglandins and the kidney. *Am J Med* 1982; **72**: 354–74.

[261] Owens MR, Cave WT. Dietary fish lipids do not diminish platelet adhesion to subendothelium. *Br J Haematol* 1990; **75**: 82–5.

[262] Li XL, Steiner M. Fish oil: a potent inhibitor of platelet adhesiveness. *Blood* 1990; **76**: 938–45.

[263] Nordoy A, Rodset JM. The influences of dietary fats on platelets in man. *Acta Med Scand* 1971; **190**: 27–34.

[264] Renaud S, Morazain R, Godsey F, *et al*. Nutrients, platelet function and composition in nine groups of French and British farmers. *Atherosclerosis* 1986; **60**: 37–48.

[265] Beswick AD, Fehily AM, Sharp DS, Renaud S, Giddings J. Long-term diet modification and platelet activity. *J Intern Med* 1991; **229**: 511–5.

[266] McDonald BE, Gerrard JM, Bruce VM, Corner EJ. Comparison of the effect of canola oil and sunflower oil on plasma lipids and lipoproteins and on in vivo thromboxane A2 and prostacyclin production in healthy young men. *Am J Clin Nutr* 1989; **50**: 1382–8.

[267] La Guarde M, Burtin M, Sprecher H, Dechavanne M, Renaud S. Potentiating effect of 5,8,11-eicosatrienoic acid on human platelet aggregation. *Lipids* 1983; **18**: 291–4.

[268] Sirtori CR, Tremoli E, Gatti E, *et al*. Controlled evaluation of fat intake in the Mediterranean diet: comparative activities of olive oil and corn oil on plasma lipids and platelets in high-risk patients. *Am J Clin Nutr* 1986; **44**: 635–42.

[269] Barradas MA, Christofides JA, Jeremy JY, Mikhailidis DP, Fry DE, Dandona P. The effect of olive oil supplementation on human platelet function, serum cholesterol-related variables and plasma fibrinogen concentration: a pilot study. *Nutr Res* 1990; **10**: 403–11.

[270] Miller GJ, Cruickshank JK, Ellis LJ, *et al*. Fat consumption and factor VII coagulant activity in middle-aged men: an association between a dietary and thrombogenic coronary risk factor. *Atherosclerosis* 1989; **78**: 19–24.

[271] Miller GJ, Martin JC, Webster J, *et al*. Association between dietary fat intake and plasma factor VII coagulant activity – a predictor of cardiovascular mortality. *Atherosclerosis* 1986; **60**: 269–77.

[272] Marckmann P, Sandstrom B, Jespersen J. Effects of total fat content and fatty acid composition in diet on factor VII coagulant activity and blood lipids. *Atherosclerosis* 1990; **80**: 227–33.

[273] Poole JC. The effect of certain fatty acids on the coagulation of plasma in vitro. *Br J Exp Pathol* 1955; **36**: 248–53.

[274] Connor WE. The acceleration of thrombus formation by certain fatty acids. *J Clin Invest* 1962; **41**: 1199–205.

[275] Miller GJ, Martin JC, Mitropoulos KA, *et al*. Plasma factor VII is activated by postprandial triglyceridaemia, irrespective of dietary fat composition. *Atherosclerosis* 1991; **86**: 163–71.

[276] Sanders TA, Vickers M, Haines AP. Effect on blood lipids and haemostasis of a supplement of cod-liver oil, rich in eicosapentaenoic and docosahexaenoic acids, in healthy young men. *Clin Sci* 1981; **61**: 317–24.

[277] Brox JH, Killie JE, Osterud B, Holme S, Nordoy A. Effects of cod liver oil on platelets and coagulation in familial hypercholesterolemia (type IIa). *Acta Med Scand* 1983; **213**: 137–44.

[278] Hostmark AT, Bjerkedal T, Kierulf P, Flaten H, Ulshagen K. Fish oil and plasma fibrinogen. *BMJ* 1988; **297**: 180–1.

[279] Hansen JB, Olsen JO, Wilsgard L, Osterud B. Effects of dietary supplementation with cod liver oil on monocyte thromboplastin synthesis, coagulation and fibrinolysis. *J Intern Med* 1989; **225** (suppl 1): 133–9.

[280] Barcelli U, Glas-Greenwalt P, Pollak VE. Enhancing effect of dietary supplementation with omega-3 fatty acids on plasma fibrinolysis in normal subjects. *Thromb Res* 1985; **39**: 307–12.

[281] Mehta J, Lawson D, Saldeen T. Reduction in plasminogen activator inhibitor-1 (PA1-1) with omega-3 polyunsaturated fatty acid (PUFA) intake. *Am Heart J* 1988; **116**: 1201–6.

[282] Schmidt EB, Ernst E, Varming K, Pedersen JO, Dyerberg J. The effect of n-3 fatty acids on lipids and haemostasis in patients with type IIa and type IV hyperlipidaemia. *Thromb Haemost* 1989; **62**: 797–801.

[283] Schmidt EB, Varming K, Ernst E, Madsen P, Dyerberg J. Dose-response studies on the effect of n-3 polyunsaturated fatty acids on lipids and haemostasis. *Thromb Haemost* 1990; **63**: 1–5.

[284] Radack K, Deck C, Huster G. Dietary supplementation with low-dose fish oils lowers fibrinogen levels: a randomized, double-blind controlled study. *Ann Intern Med* 1989; **111**: 757–8.

[285] Takimoto G, Galang J, Lee GK, Bradlow BA. Plasma fibrolytic activity after ingestion of omega-3 fatty acids in human subjects. *Thromb Res* 1989; **54**: 573–82.

[286] Mehrabian M, Peter JB, Barnard RJ, Lusis AJ. Dietary regulation of fibrinolytic factors. *Atherosclerosis* 1990; **84**: 25–32.

[287] Bonaa KH, Bjerve KS, Straume B, Gram IT, Thelle D. Effect of eicosapentanenoic acid and docosahexanenoic acid on blood pressure in hypertension. A population based intervention trial from the Tromso Study. *N Engl J Med* 1990; **322**: 795–801.

[288] British Nutrition Foundation. *Unsaturated fatty acids: nutritional and physiological significance: the report of the British Nutrition Foundation's Task Force*. London: Chapman & Hall for the British Nutrition Foundation, 1992.

[289] Rogers S, James KS, Butland BK, Etherington MD, O'Brien JR, Jones JG. Effects of a fish oil supplement on serum lipids, blood pressure, bleeding time, haemostatic and rheological variables. A double-blind randomised controlled trial in healthy volunteers. *Atherosclerosis* 1987; **63**: 137–43.

[290] Van Houwelingen R, Nordoy A, Van der Beek E, Houtsmuller U, de Metz M, Hornstra G. Effect of a moderate fish intake on blood pressure, bleeding times, haematology and clinical chemistry in healthy males. *Am J Clin Nutr* 1987; **46**: 424–36.

291 Cobiac L, Nestel P, wing LMH, Howe PRC. The effects of dietary sodium restriction and fish oils supplements in the elderly. *Clin Exp Pharmacol Physiol* 1991; **18**: 265–8.

[292] Grundy SM. Comparison of monounsaturated fatty acids and carbohydrates for lowering plasma cholesterol. *N Engl J Med* 1986; **314**: 745–48.

[293] Lewis B, Hammett F, Katan M, *et al*. Towards an improved lipid-lowering diet: additive effects of changes in nutrient intake. *Lancet* 1981; **2**: 1310–3.

[294] Rosenthal MB, Barnard RJ, Rose DP, Inkeles S, Hall J, Pritikin N. Effects of a high-complex-carbohydrate, low-fat, low-cholesterol diet on levels of serum lipids and estradiol. *Am J Med* 1985; **78**: 23–7.

[295] Weisweiler P, Janetschek P, Schwandt P. Influence of polyunsaturated fats and fat restriction on serum lipoproteins in humans. *Metabolism* 1985; **34**: 83–7.

[296] Jenkins DJ. Carbohydrates: (B) dietary fibre. In: Shils ME, Young VR, eds. *Modern nutrition in health and disease*. 7th ed. Philadelphia: Lea & Febiger, 1988; 52–71.

[297] Kromhout D, Bosschieter EB, de Lezenne Coulander C. Dietary fibre and 10-year mortality from coronary heat disease, cancer and all causes: the Zutphen study. *Lancet* 1982; **ii**: 518–22.

[298] Ripsin CM, Keenan JM, Jacobs DR, Elmer PJ, Welch RR et al. Oat products and lipid lowering: A meta-analysis. *JAMA* 1992; **267**: 3317–3325.

[299] Morris JN, Marr JW, Clayton DG. Diet and heart: a postscript. *BMJ* 1977; **2**: 1307–14.

[300] Yano K, Rhoads GG, Kagan A, Tillotson J. Dietary intake and risk of coronary heart disease in Japanese men living in Hawaii. *Am J Clin Nutr* 1978; **31**: 1270–9.

[301] Gey KF, Puska P, Jordan P, Moser UK. Inverse correlation between plasma vitamin E and mortality from ischemic heart disease in cross-cultural epidemiology. *Am J Clin Nutr* 1991; **53** (1 Suppl): 326S–34S.

[302] Riemersma RA, Wood DA, Macintyre CC, Elton RA, Gey KF, Oliver MF. Risk of angina pectoris and plasma concentrations of vitamins A, C, and E and carotene. *Lancet* 1991; **337**: 1–5.

[303] Rimm EB, Stampfer MJ, Ascherio A, Giovanuucci E, Colditz GA, Willett WC. Vitamin E consumption and the risk of coronary heart disease in men. *N Engl J Med* 1993; **328**: 1450–6.

[304] Stampfer MJ, Hennekens CH, Manson JE, Colditz GA, Rosner B, Willett WC. Vitamin E consumption and the risk of coronary disease in women. *N Engl J Med* 1993; **328**: 1444–9.

[305] Hertog MG, Feskens EJ, Hollman PC, Katan MB, Kromhout D. Dietary antioxidant flavonoids and risk of coronary heart disease: the Zutphen Elderly Study. *Lancet* 1993; **342**: 1007–11.

[306] Salonen JT, Yla-Herttuala S, Yamamoto R, *et al*. Autoantibody against oxidised LDL and progression of carotid atherosclerosis. *Lancet* 1992; **339**: 883–7.

[307] Regnstrom J, Nilsson J, Tornvall P, Landou C, Hamsten A. Susceptibility to low-density lipoprotein oxidation and coronary atherosclerosis in man. *Lancet* 1992; **339**: 1183–6.

[308] Bonanome A, Pagnan A, Biffanti S, Opportuno A, Sorgato F, Dorella M, Maiorino M, Ursini F. Effect of dietary monounsaturated and polyunsaturated fatty acids on the susceptibility of plasma low density lipoproteins to oxidative modification. *Arterioscler Thromb* 1992; **12**: 529–533.

[309] Esterbauer H, Rotheneder M, Striegl G, *et al*. Vitamin E and other lipophilic antioxidants protect LDL against oxidation. *Fat Science Technology* 1989; **91**: 316–24.

[310] Frei B. Ascorbic acid protects lipids in human plasma and low-density lipoprotein against oxidative damage. *Am J Clin Nutr* 1991; **54** (6 Suppl): 1113S–8S.

[311] Sarkkinen ES, Uusitupa MIJ, Nyyssonen K, Parviainen M, Penttila I, Salonen JT. Effects of two low fat diets, high and low in polyunsaturated fatty acids, on plasma lipid peroxides and serum vitamin E levels in free-living hypercholesterolaemic men. *Eur J Clin Nutr* 1993; **47**: 623–30.

[312] Ascherio A, Willet WC. Are body iron stores related to the risk of coronary heart disease? *New Eng J Med* 1994; **330**: 1152–1154.

[313] Salonen JT, Nyyssonen K, Korpela H, Tuomilehto J, Seppanen R, Salonen R. High stored iron levels are associated with excess risk of myocardial infarction in eastern Finnish men. *Circulation* 1992; **86**: 803–11.

[314] Morrison HI, Semenciw RM, Mao Y, Wigle DT. Serum iron and risk of fatal acute myocardial infarction. *Epidemiology* 1994; **5**: 243–6.

[315] Stampfer MJ, Grodstein F, Rosenberg I, Willet W, Hennekens C. A prospective study of plasma ferritin and risk of myocardial infarction in US physicians. *Circulation* 1993; **87**: 688 (abstract).

[316] Magnusson MK, Sigfusson N, Sigraldasin H, Johannesson GM, Magnusson S, Thorgeirsson G. Low iron binding capacity as a risk factor for myocardial infarction. *Circulation* 1994; **89**: 102–8.

[317] Sempos CT, Looker AC, Gillum RF, Makuc DM. Body iron stores and the risk of coronary heart disease. *New Eng J Med* 1994; **330**: 1119–24.

[318] Ascherio A, Willett WC, Rimm EB, Giovannucci EL, Stampfer MJ. Dietary iron intake and risk of coronary disease among men. *Circulation* 1991; **89**: 969–974.

[319] Steinberg D. Antioxidant vitamins and coronary heart disease. *N Engl J Med* 1993; **328**: 1487–9.

[320] The Alpha-Tocopherol, Beta Carotene Cancer Prevention Study Group. The effect of vitamin E and beta carotene on the incidence of lung cancer and other cancers in male smokers. *New Eng J Med* 1994; **330**: 1029–35.

[321] Dahl LK. Salt and hypertension. *Am J Clin Nutr* 1972; **25**: 231–44.

[322] Morgan T, Anderson A. Sodium restriction can delay the return of hypertension in patients previously well-controlled on drug therapy. *Can J Physiol Pharmacol* 1987; **65**: 1752–5.

[323] Weinberger MH, Cohen SJ, Miller JZ, Luft FC, Grim CE, Fineberg NS. Dietary sodium restriction as adjunctive treatment of hypertension. *JAMA* 1988; **259**: 2561–5.

[324] MacGregor GA, Markandu ND, Sagnella GA, Singer DR, Cappuccio FP. Double-blind study of three sodium intakes and long-term effects of sodium restriction in essential hypertension. *Lancet* 1989; **2**: 1244–7.

[325] Sullivan JM, Ratts TE, Taylor JC, *et al*. Hemodynamic effects of dietary sodium in man: a preliminary report. *Hypertension* 1980; **2**: 506–14.

[326] Parfrey PS, Markandu ND, Roulston JE, Jones BE, Jones JC, MacGregor GA. Relation between arterial pressure, dietary sodium intake, and renin system in essential hypertension. *BMJ* 1981; **283**: 94–7.

[327] Stokes GS, Monaghan JC, Middleton AT, Shirlow M, Marwood JF. Effects of dietary sodium deprivation on erythrocyte sodium concentration and cation transport in normotensive and untreated hypertensive subjects. *J Hypertens* 1986; **4**: 35–8.

[328] Muntzel M, Drueke T. A comprehensive review of the salt and blood pressure relationship. *Am J Hypertens* 1992; **5**(4 Pt 1): 1S–42S.

[329] Intersalt Cooperative Research Group. Intersalt: an international study of electrolyte excretion and blood pressure. Results for 24 hour urinary sodium and potassium excretion. *BMJ* 1988; **297**: 319–28.

[330] Elliott P, Dyer A, Stamler R, Stamler J. Correcting for regression dilution in INTERSALT. *Lancet* 1993; **342**: 1123.

[331] Law MR, Frost CD, Wald NJ. By how much does dietary salt reduction lower blood pressure? I–III – Analysis of observational data among populations. *BMJ* 1991; **302**: 811–5; 815–19; 819–24.

[332] Swales JD. Dietary salt and blood pressure: the role of meta-analyses. *J Hypertens* 1991; **9**(suppl 6): S42–6.

[333] Law MR, Frost CD, Wald NJ. Dietary salt and blood pressure. *J Hypertens* 1991; **9**(suppl 6): S37–41.

[334] Cappuccio FP, MacGregor GA. Does potassium supplementation lower blood pressure? A meta-analysis of published trials. *J Hypertens* 1991; **9**: 465–73.

[335] Sanchez-Castillo CP, Warrender S, Whitehead TP, James WP. An assessment of the sources of dietary salt in a British population. *Clin Sci* 1987; **72**: 95–102

[336] Larsen HN. Sensory and technological aspects of sodium chloride reduction and partial replacement with potassium chloride in white bread. Bread Research Institute of Australia. Sydney 1993.

[337] Marmot M, Brunner E. Alcohol and cardiovascular disease: the status of the U-shaped curve. *BMJ* 1991; **303**: 565–8.

[338] Health Update No 3: Alcohol. Health Education Authority. London, 1993.

[339] Marmot MG, Rose G, Shipley MJ, Thomas BJ. Alcohol and mortality: a U-shaped curve. *Lancet* 1981; **1**: 580–3.

[340] Royal College of Physicians. A great and growing evil: the medical consequences of alcohol abuse. London: Tavistock, 1987.

[341] Klatsky AL. Blood pressure and alcohol consumption. In: Bulpitt CJ, ed. *Epidemiology of hypertension*. Amsterdam: Elsevier, 1985: 159–74. (Birkenhäger WH, Reid JL, eds. Handbook of hypertension; vol 6).

[342] Klatsky AL, Friedman GD, Armstrong MA. The relationships between alcoholic beverage use and other traits to blood pressure: a new Kaiser Permanente study. *Circulation* 1986; **73**: 628–36.

[343] Dyer AR, Stamler J, Paul O, *et al*. Alcohol consumption, cardiovascular risk factors, and mortality in two Chicago epidemiologic studies. *Circulation* 1977; **56**: 1067–74.

[344] Camargo CA. Moderate alcohol consumption and stroke: the epidemiologic evidence. *Stroke* 1989; **20**: 1611–26.

[345] Hillbom M, Kaste M. Ethanol intoxication: a risk factor for ischemic brain infarction. *Stroke* 1983; **14**: 694–9.

[346] Stampfer MJ, Colditz GA, Willett WC, Speizer FE, Hennekens CH. A prospective study of moderate alcohol consumption and the risk of coronary disease and stroke in women. *N Engl J Med* 1988; **319**: 267–73.

[347] St Leger AS, Cochrane AL, Moore F. Factors associated with cardiac mortality in developed countries with particular reference to the consumption of wine. *Lancet* 1979; **1**: 1017–20.

[348] Boffetta P, Garfinkel L. Alcohol drinking and mortality among men enrolled in an American Cancer Society prospective study. *Epidemiology* 1990; **1**: 342–8.

[349] Rimm EB, Giovannucci EL, Willett WC *et al*. Prospective study of alcohol consumption and risk of coronary disease in men. *Lancet* 1991; **338**: 464–8.

[350] Hegsted DM, Ausman LM. Diet, alcohol and coronary heart disease in men. *J Nutr* 1988; **118**: 1184–9.

[351] Shaper AG. Alcohol and mortality: a review of prospective studies. *Br J Addict* 1990; **85**: 837–47.

[352] Klatsky AL, Armstrong MA, Friedman GD. Alcohol and cardiovascular deaths. *Circulation* 1989; **80**: (4 Suppl II): II–614 (abstract 2438).

[353] Klatsky AL, Armstrong MA, Friedman GD. Mortality in ex-drinkers. *Circulation* 1990; **81**: 720 (abstract 34).

[354] Kono S, Ikeda M, Ogata M, Tokudome S, Nishizumi M, Kuratsune M. The relationship between alcohol and mortality among Japanese physicians. *Int J Epidemiol* 1983; **12**: 437–41.

[355] Yano K, Rhoads GG, Kagan A. Coffee, alcohol and risk of coronary heart disease among Japanese men living in Hawaii. *N Engl J Med* 1977; **297**: 405–9.

[356] Jackson R, Scragg R, Beaglehole R. Alcohol consumption and the risk of coronary heart disease. *BMJ* 1991; **303**: 211–6.

[357] Lazarus NB, Kaplan GA, Cohen RD, Leu DJ. Change in alcohol consumption and risk of death from all causes and from ischaemic heart disease. *BMJ* 1991; **303**: 553–6.

[358] Gaziano JM, Buring JE, Breslow JL, Goldhaber SZ, Rosner B, Vandenburgh M, Willett WC, Hennekens CH. Moderate alcohol intake, increased levels of high density lipoprotein and its subfractions, and decreased risk of myocardial infarction. *New Eng J Med* 1993; **329**: 1829–34.

[359] Castelli WP, Doyle JT, Gordon T, *et al*. Alcohol and blood lipids: the Cooperative Lipoprotein Phenotyping Study. *Lancet* 1977; **2**: 153–5.

[360] Criqui MH, Cowan LD, Tyroler HA, *et al*. Lipoproteins as mediators for the effects of alcohol consumption and cigarette smoking on cardiovascular mortality: results from the Lipids Research Clinics follow-up study. *Am J Epidemiol* 1987; **126**: 629–37.

[361] Meade TW, Chakrabarti R, Haines AP, North WR, Stirling Y. Characteristics affecting fibrinolytic activity and plasma fibrinogen concentrations. *BMJ* 1979; **1**: 153–6.

[362] Renaud SC, Beswick AD, Fehily AM, Sharp DS, Elwood PC. Alcohol and platelet aggregation, the Caerphilly Prospective Heart Disease Study. *Am J Clin Nutr* 1992; **55**: 1012–7.

[363] Frankel EN, Kanner J, German JB, Parks E, Kinsella JE. Inhibition of oxidation of human low density lipoprotein by phenolic substances in red wine. *Lancet* 1993; **341**: 454–7.

[364] Rose G, Day S. The population mean predicts the number of deviant individuals. *BMJ* 1990; **301**: 1031–4.

[365] Duffy JC. Fallacy of the distribution of alcohol consumption. *Psychol Rep* 1982; **50**: 125–6.

[366] Royal College of Physicians. Obesity: a report of the Royal College of Physicians. *J R Coll Physicians Lond*, 1983; **17**: 5–65.

[367] Saad MF, Lillioja S, Nyombu BL, Castillo C, Ferraro R, de Gregario M, Ravussin E, Knowler WC, Bennett PH, Howard BV, Bogardus C. Racial differences in the relation between blood pressure and insulin resistance. *New Eng J Med* 1991; **324**: 733–739.

[368] Romieu I, Willett WC, Stampfer MJ, et al. Energy intake and other determinants of relative weight. *Am J Clin Nutr* 1988; **47**: 406–12.

[369] Kromhout D. Energy and macronutrient intake in lean and obese middle-aged men (the Zutphen study). *Am J Clin Nutr* 1983; **37**: 295–9.

[370] Baecke JA, Van Staveren WA, Burema J. Food composition, habitual physical activity and body fatness in young Dutch adults. *Am J Clin Nutr* 1983; **37**: 278–86.

[371] Flatt JP. The biochemistry of energy expenditure. In: Bray GA, ed. *Recent advances in obesity research II: proceedings of the 2nd international congress on obesity, 23–26 October 1977, Washington DC*. London: Newman, 1978; 211–28.

[372] Dreon DM, Frey-Hewitt B, Ellsworth N, Williams PT, Terry RB, Wood PD. Dietary fat:carbohydrate ratio and obesity in middle-aged men. *Am J Clin Nutr* 1988; **47**: 995–1000.

[373] Lissner L, Levitsky DA, Strupp BJ, Kalkwarf HJ, Roe DA. Dietary fat and the regulation of energy intake in human subjects. *Am J Clin Nutr* 1987; **46**: 886–92.

[374] Stubbs RJ, Murgatroyd PR, Goldberg GR, Prentice AM. The effect of covert manipulation of dietary fat and energy density on ad lib. food intake in humans. *Proc Nut Soc* 1993; **52**: 35A (abstract).

[375] Stubbs RJ, Ritz P, Coward WA, Prentice AM. The effect of covert manipulation of dietary fat and energy density on ad lib food intake in "free-living" humans. *Proc Nut Soc* 1993: **52**:348A (abstract).

[376] Stubbs RJ, Prentice AM. The effect of covertly manipulating the dietary fat:carbohydrate ratio of isoenergetically dense diets on ad lib food intake in "free-living" humans. *Proc Nut Soc* 1993;**52**:551A (abstract).

[377] Lawton CL, Burley VJ, Wales JK, Blundell JE. Dietary fat and appetite control in obese subjects: weak effects on satiation and satiety. *Int J Obes* 1993; **17**: 409–16.

[378] Blundell J, Burley V, Cotton J, Lawton C. Dietary fat and appetite control: weak effects on satiation (within-meals) and satiety (following-meals). In: Mela DJ, ed. *Dietary fats: determinants of preference, selection and consumption*. London: Elsevier Applied Science, 1992; 79–101.

172

[379] Flatt JP, Ravussin E, Acheson KJ, Jequier E. Effects of dietary fat on postprandial substrate oxidation and on carbohydrate and fat balances. *J Clin Invest* 1985; **76**: 1019–24.

[380] Flatt JP. Dietary fat, carbohydrate balance and weight maintenance: effects of exercise. *Am J Clin Nutr* 1987; **45**: 296–306.

[381] Stubbs RJ, Murgatroyd PR, Goldberg GR, Prentice AM. Carbohydrate balance and the regulation of day-to-day food intake in humans. *Am J Clin Nutr* 1993; **57**: 897–903.

[382] LaCroix AZ, Mead LA, Liang KY, Thomas CB, Pearson TA. Coffee consumption and the incidence of coronary heart disease. *N Engl J Med* 1986; **315**: 977–82.

[383] Grobbee DE, Rimm EB, Giovannucci E, Colditz G, Stampfer M, Willett W. Coffee, caffeine and cardiovascular disease in men. *N Engl J Med* 1990; **323**: 1026–32.

[384] LeGrady D, Dyer AR, Shekelle RB, *et al*. Coffee consumption and mortality in the Chicago Western Electric Company Study. *Am J Epidemiol* 1987; **126**: 803–12.

[385] Tverdal A, Stensvold I, Solvoll K, Foss OP, Lund-Larsen P, Bjartveit K. Coffee consumption and death from coronary heart disease in middle-aged Norweigan men and women. *BMJ* 1990; **300**: 566–9.

[386] Bak AA, Grobbee DE. The effect on serum cholesterol levels of coffee brewed by filtering or boiling. *N Engl J Med* 1989; **321**: 1432–7.

[387] Zock PL, Katan MB, Merkus MP, van Dusseldorp M, Harryvan JL. Effect of a lipid rich fraction from boiled coffee on serum cholesterol. *Lancet* 1990; **335**: 1235–7.

[388] Brown CA, Bolton-Smith C, Woodward M, Tunstall-Pedoe H. Coffee and tea consumption and the prevalence of coronary heart disease in men and women: results from the Scottish Heart Health Study. *J Epidemiol Community Health* 1993; **47**: 171–5.

[389] Clarke R, Daly L, Robinson K, *et al*. Hyperhomocysteinemia: an independent risk factor for vascular disease. *N Engl J Med* 1991; **324**: 1149–55

[390] Daly L, Robinson K, Tan KS, Graham IM. Hyperhomocysteinaemia: a metabolic risk factor for coronary heart disease determined by both genetic and environmental influences? *Q J Med* 1993; **86**: 685–9.

[391] Kleijnen J, Knipschild P, ter Riet G. Garlic, onions and cardiovascular risk factors: a review of the evidence from human experiments with emphasis on commercially available preparations. *Br J Clin Pharmacol* 1989; **28**: 535–44.

[392] Mansell P and Reckless JP. Garlic: effects on serum lipids, blood pressure, coagulation, platelet aggregation and vasodilation. *BMJ* 1991; **303**: 379–80.

[393] Strong JP, Newman WP, Freedman DS, Gard PD, Tracy RE, Solberg LA. Atherosclerotic disease in children and young adults: relation to cardiovascular risk factors. In: Berenson GS, ed. *Causation of cardiovascular risk factors in children: perspectives on cardiovascular risk in early life*. New York: Raven Press, 1986; 27–41.

[394] American Academy of Paediatrics. Committee on Nutrition. Prudent life-style for children: dietary fat and cholesterol. *Pediatrics* 1986; **78**: 521–5.

[395] Berenson GS, Voors AW, Gard P, Newman WP, Tracy RE. Clinical and anatomical correlates of cardiovascular disease in children from the Bogalusa Heart Study. In: Schettler FG, *et al*, eds. *Atherosclerosis VI*. Berlin: Springer-Verlag; 1982; 60–65.

[396] Webber LS, Srinivasan SR, Wattingey WA, Berenson GS. Tracking of serum lipids and lipoproteins from childhood to adulthood: the Bogalusa Heart Study. *Am J Epidemiol* 1991; **133**: 884–99.

[397] Lauer RM, Lee J, Clarke WR. Factors affecting the relationship between childhood and adult cholesterol levels: the Muscatine Study. *Pediatrics* 1988; **82**: 309–18.

[398] Boulton TJ, Magarey A, Cockington R. Cholesterol from infancy to age thirteen: tracking and parent-child associations. *Ann Nestlé* 1990; **48**: 70–6.

[399] Report of the National Cholesterol Education Program Expert Panel on Detection, Evaluation and Treatment of High Blood Cholesterol in Adults. *Arch Int Med* 1988; **148**: 36–69.

[400] Department of Health and Social Security. *Present day practice in infant feeding: third report: report of a Working Party of the Panel on Child Nutrition, Committee on Medical Aspects of Food Policy*. London: HMSO, 1988.(Report on Health and Social Subjects; 32).

[401] World Health Organisation. Collaborative study on breast feeding. *The quantity and quality of breast milk: report on the WHO collaborative study on breast-feeding*. Geneva: WHO, 1985.

[402] Casey CE, Hambidge KM. Nutritional aspect of human lactation. In: Neville MC, Neifert MR, eds. *Lactation: physiology, nutrition and breast-feeding*. New York: Plenum, 1983: 199–248.

[403] Department of Health and Social Security. *The composition of mature human milk: report of a Working Party of the Committee on Medical Aspects of Food Policy*. London: HMSO, 1977.(Report on Health and Social Subjects; 12).

[404] Department of Health and Social Security. *A nutrition survey of pre-school children 1967–68: report by the Committee on Medical Aspects of Food Policy*. London: HMSO, 1975. (Report on Health and Social Subjects; 10).

[405] Beauchamp GK. Ontogenesis of taste preferences. In: Walcher DN, Kretchmer N, eds. *Food, nutrition and evolution: food as an environmental factor in the genesis of human variability*. New York: Masson, 1981: 49–57.

[406] Yeung DL, Pennell MD, Leung M, Hall J. The effects of 2% milk intake on infant nutrition. *Nutr Res* 1982; **2**: 651–60.

[407] Hagman U, Bruce A, Persson L, Samuelson G, Sjolin S. Food habits and nutrient intake in childhood in relation to health and socio-economic conditions: a Swedish multicentre study 1980–81. *Acta Paediatr Scand* 1986; Suppl 328: 4–56.

[408] Barrett-Connor E, Suarez L, Khaw KT, Criqui MH, Wingard DL. Ischaemic heart disease risk factors after age 50. *J Chron Dis* 1984; **37**: 903–8.

[409] Stamler J, Wentworth D, Neaton JD. Is the relationship between serum cholesterol and risk of premature death from coronary heart disease continuous and graded? Findings in 356 222 primary screenees of the Multiple Risk Factor Intervention Trial (MRFIT). *JAMA* 1986; **256**: 2823–8.

[410] Aronson MK, Ooi WL, Morgenstern PH *et al*. Women, myocardial infarction and dementia in the very old. *Neurology* 1990; **40**: 1102–6.

[411] Shipley MJ, Pocock SJ, Marmot MG. Does plasma cholesterol concentration predict mortality from coronary heart disease in elderly people? 18 year follow-up in Whitehall study. *BMJ* 1991; **303**: 89–92.

[412] Manolio TA, Pearson TA, Wenger NK, Barrett-Connor E, Payne GH, Harlan WR. Cholesterol and heart disease in older persons and women. Review of an NHLBI Workshop. *Ann Epidemiol* 1992; **2**: 161–176.

[413] Gordon DJ, Rifkind BM. Treating high blood cholesterol in the older patient. *Am J Cardiol* 1989; **63**: 48H–52H.

[414] Department of Health. *The Nutrition of Elderly People*. London: HMSO, 1992. (Report on Health and Social Subjects; 43).

10. Glossary

Atherosclerosis disease of the arteries, including those supplying the heart muscle, in which fatty fibrous plaques develop on the inner walls of the artery.

Apoprotein the protein moiety of lipoproteins

Blood pressure the pulsating pressure of blood on the walls of main arteries: systolic pressure, or highest pressure, occurs when the heart is contracting and diastolic, or lowest pressure, when it is relaxing

BMI Body Mass Index = $\dfrac{\text{weight (kg)}}{\text{height(m)}^2}$

Cardiovascular relating to the heart and blood vessels

DRV Dietary Reference Value

Double bond a chemical bond between 2 carbon atoms in a fatty acid formed by the sharing of 2 pairs of electrons

EFA essential fatty acid; one which cannot be made in the body but which must be supplied by food (linoleic acid or α-linolenic acid)

Embolus material, such as a thrombus or a foreign body, that is carried by the blood from one point in the circulation to another where it lodges

Extrinsic sugars sugars not located within the cellular structure of a food, eg table sugar, honey

Fat see triglycerides

Fibrinolysis the process by which the fibrin mesh of blood clots and thrombi is dissolved

HDL high density lipoprotein

Hydrogenated fat soft or liquid fat which has been hardened by the addition of hydrogen using a catalyst

Incidence number of new events (eg reports of a disease) arising in defined units of the population and time (often 1 year)

ICD International Classification of Diseases (WHO)

Intrinsic sugars sugars naturally present and embodied in the cellular structure of a food, eg sugars in an orange

kcal kilocalorie (1 thousand calories); a unit of food energy

kJ kilojoule (1 thousand joules); a unit of food energy (1 kcal = 4.184 kJ)

Lipoproteins	lipid-protein complexes in which cholesterol, triglycerides and other substances are transported in the blood
LDL	low density lipoprotein
MJ	megajoule (1 million joules)
mmol	millimole; amount of substance; 1 millimole = molecular weight in milligrams
MONICA	Multinational monitoring of trends and determinants in cardiovascular disease (A WHO project)
Monounsaturates	monounsaturated fatty acids (MUFA); fatty acids with one double (unsaturated) bond
Morbidity	ill health due to disease
Mortality rate	total number of persons dying of a disease in relation to defined units of the population and time.
NSP	non-starch polysaccharides; a precisely measurable and major component of dietary fibre
Obesity	BMI over 30 kg/m^2
Overweight	BMI 25–30 kg/m^2
Phospholipids	lipids which contain phosphorus; generally composed of 2 fatty acids and 1 phosphate attached to a glycerol backbone; important components of cell membranes
Polyunsaturates	polyunsaturated fatty acids (PUFA); fatty acids with 2 or more double (unsaturated) bonds
Prevalence	the occurrence of a disease or condition described as the total number of persons with that condition in a defined unit of the population at any particular time
Prostaglandins	a group of substances derived from 20-carbon polyunsaturated fatty acids; potent mediators of a wide range of metabolic processes (*qv* thromboxanes)
Saturates	Saturated fatty acids (SFA); fatty acids with carbon atoms fully saturated with hydrogen, ie with no double bonds
Thrombosis	development or presence of a thrombus
Thromboxanes	a group of substances derived from 20-carbon polyunsaturated fatty acids; potent mediators of vasoconstriction and platelet aggregation (*qv* prostaglandins)
Thrombus	the result of platelet activation and aggregation associated with activation of the blood clotting system; a fibrin-rich mesh containing copious platelets
Triglycerides	lipid esters composed of 3 fatty acid molecules joined to 1 molecule of glycerol; triglycerides constitute the major part of dietary fat
VLDL	very low density lipoprotein
WHO	World Health Organisation

Appendix A *Percentage distribution of serum total cholesterol by age and sex in England*

Total cholesterol (mmol/l)	Age							Total
	18-24	25-34	35-44	45-54	55-64	65-74	75 and over	
	%	%	%	%	%	%	%	%
Men								
Less than 5.2	66	48	28	17	19	16	23	31
5.2 – less than 6.5	30	38	49	46	46	43	41	43
6.5 – less than 7.8	2	13	19	29	29	36	36	23
7.8 or more	3	1	4	7	6	5	–	4
Base	108	219	210	177	148	129	86	1077
Women								
Less than 5.2	70	51	43	17	7	4	7	30
5.2 – less than 6.5	24	40	43	50	38	32	37	39
6.5 – less than 7.8	6	8	13	26	41	35	42	23
7.8 or more	–	1	2	8	14	28	14	9
Base	101	236	229	187	164	145	102	1164

Source: White *et al*, 1992[27]

Figures B.1–B.4 cover the whole period 1951 to 1990 for England and Wales. Figures B.3 + B.4 show the trends in more detail for those aged 35–64. In the period up to 1967, particularly from the mid 1950s to mid 1960s, death rates for CHD for males under 65 rose, while those in the older age-groups fell, giving little overall change. In the last decade, however, there have been sharp falls in CHD death rates in the younger age-groups and some decline in the older groups producing a fall in the rate for all ages. For females, there were sharp falls in

Figure B.1 Standardised mortality rates[†] for coronary heart disease by sex and age (all ages over and under 65 years), England and Wales, 1950-1991*

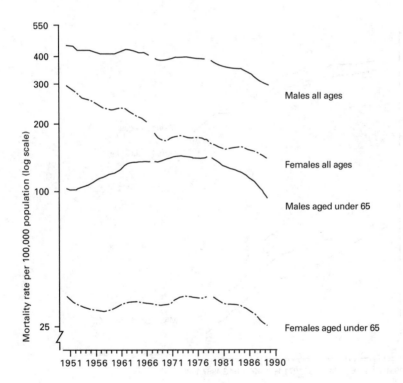

[†] Rates are calculated using the European Standard Population with a 3 year average plotted against middle of average

* There are discontinuities due to a change from ICD 7 to ICD 8 in 1968 and from ICD 8 to ICD 9 in 1979.

In 1984, there was a change in the rule affecting the classification of the major and underlying causes of death - this may also affect comparisons.

CHD death rates in the older age-groups in the 1950s and smaller falls or little change in the younger groups resulting in an overall fall; more recently, as for males, the falls have been greater in the younger age-groups. There was little change in overall male death rates for stroke until the early 1960s after which they fell, accelerating somewhat in recent years. The fall has been greater among the under 65s than in older age-groups. For women the pattern of stroke deaths has been similar but with a slightly greater fall overall and particularly among the under 65s.

Figure B.2 Standardised mortality rates[†] for stroke by sex and age (all ages and under 65 years) England and Wales 1950-1991*

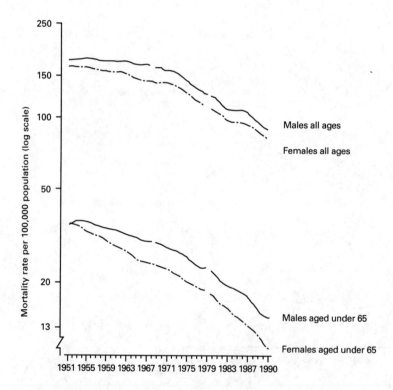

[†] Rates are calculated using the European Standard Population with a 3 year average plotted against middle of average

* There are discontinuities due to a change from ICD 7 to ICD 8 in 1968 and from ICD 8 to ICD 9 in 1979.

In 1984, there was a change in the rule affecting the classification of the major and underlying causes of death - this may also affect comparisons.

180

Figure B.3 Standardised mortality rates[†] for coronary heart disease by sex and age (35-64 years), England and Wales, 1950-1991*

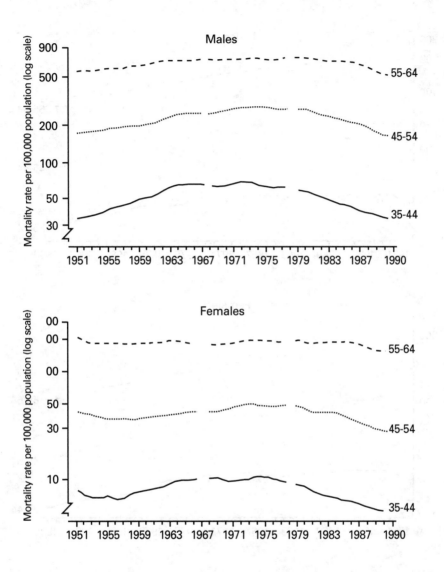

[†] Rates are calculated using the European Standard Population with a 3 year average plotted against middle of average

* There are discontinuities due to a change from ICD 7 to ICD 8 in 1968 and from ICD 8 to ICD 9 in 1979.

In 1984, there was a change in the rule affecting the classification of the major and underlying causes of death - this may also affect comparisons.

Figure B.4 Standardised mortality rates † for stroke by sex and age (35-64 years), England and Wales, 1950-1991*

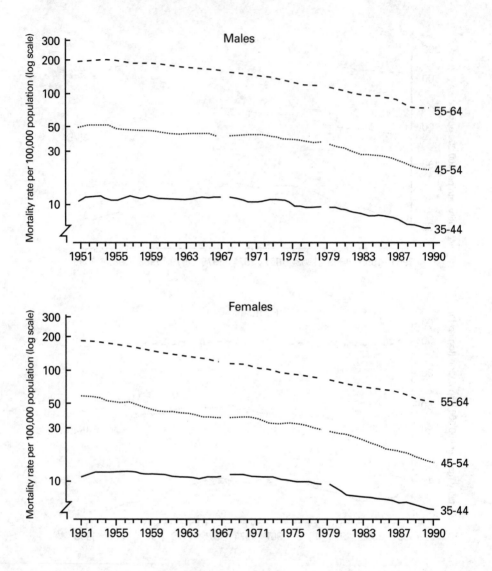

† Rates are calculated using the European Standard Population with a 3 year average plotted against middle of average

* There are discontinuities due to a change from ICD 7 to ICD 8 in 1968 and from ICD 8 to ICD 9 in 1979.

In 1984, there was a change in the rule affecting the classification of the major and underlying causes of death - this may also affect comparisons.

Appendix C

Table C.1 The mean energy (excluding alcohol) and nutrients of the diets of average households in Great Britain 1950–1990, expressed as the amount per person per day, and the percentage of food energy supplied by protein, fat and carbohydrate.

	Energy (MJ)	Energy (kJal)	Fat (g)	Fatty acids Saturated (g)	Mono-un-saturated (g)	Poly-un-saturated (g)	P/S Ratio	Protein Total (g)	Animal (g)	Vegetable (g)	Carbo-hydrate (g)	NSP (g)	% energy from Fat	Protein	Carbo-hydrate
1950	10.3	2,474	101					78	38	40	314		36.7	12.6	50.7
1951	10.3	2,465	97					77	37	40	321		35.4	12.5	52.2
1952	10.2	2,447	94					77	38	39	324		34.5	12.6	52.9
1953	10.5	2,520	101					78	40	38	325		36.0	12.4	51.6
1954	11.0	2,626	107					77	41	36	340		36.5	11.7	51.8
1955	11.1	2,641	107					77	42	35	342		36.6	11.6	51.7
1956	11.1	2,660	111					75.1	42.7	32.4	364		37.4	11.3	51.2
1957	11.0	2,620	113					74.1	42.7	31.4	351		38.7	11.3	50.1
1958	11.0	2,630	114					74.1	42.7	31.9	351		38.5	11.3	50.0
1959	11.0	2,620	113	53.0	43.0	9.2	0.17	73.2	42.7	30.5	350		38.8	11.2	50.1
1960	11.0	2,630	115					74.7	44.1	30.6	345		39.3	11.4	49.3
1961	11.0	2,630	116					75.1	44.9	30.2	343		39.6	11.4	49.0
1962	11.1	2,640	117					73.3	45.7	29.6	342		40.0	11.4	48.6
1963	11.1	2,650	118					76.5	46.0	30.5	343		39.8	11.5	48.5
1964	10.9	2,600	116					75.1	45.1	30.0	333		40.3	11.6	48.0
1965	10.8	2,590	116					75.2	45.5	29.7	332		40.4	11.6	47.9
1966	10.7	2,560	117					75.6	46.3	29.3	321		41.0	11.8	47.0
1967	10.8	2,590	119					75.8	46.7	29.1	324		41.3	11.7	47.0
1968	10.7	2,560	118					75.4	46.6	28.8	318		41.6	11.8	46.6
1969	10.8	2,570	120	56.7	46.5	11.0	0.19	74.4	46.5	27.9	317		42.0	11.6	46.3

| | | | | Fatty acids | | | | Protein | | | Carbo-hydrate | NSP | % energy from | | Carbo- |
| | Energy | Energy | Fat | Saturated | Mono-un-saturated | Poly-un-saturated | P/S | Total | Animal | Vegetable | | | Fat | Protein | hydrate |
	(MJ)	(kjal)	(g)	(g)	(g)	(g)	Ratio	(g)	(g)	(g)	(g)	(g)			
1970	10.7	2,560	119					73.7	45.5	28.2	317		41.8	11.5	46.5
1971	10.4	2,490	117					72.4	45.1	27.3	305		42.3	11.6	46.0
1972	10.2	2,430	112	52.0	42.9	11.5	0.22	72.5	44.7	27.8	301		41.5	11.9	46.4
1973	10.0	2,400	111	51.5	41.9	11.5	0.22	71.4	44.5	26.9	293		42.0	12.0	46.0
1974	9.7	2,320	106	50.7	39.8	10.6	0.20	70.9	44.8	26.1	287		41.3	12.3	46.4
1975	9.6	2,290	107	51.7	39.8	10.1	0.19	72.0	45.8	26.1	275		42.2	12.6	45.2
1976	9.6	2,280	105	50.1	39.7	10.5	0.20	72.3	46.0	26.0	277		41.7	12.7	45.7
1977	9.5	2,260	105	47.5	39.0	10.4	0.21	72.6	46.3	26.0	273		41.9	12.8	45.3
1978	9.5	2,250	106	47.2	39.3	10.6	0.22	73.4	46.3	26.3	272		42.0	12.9	45.1
1979	9.5	2,250	106	47.8	39.7	10.7	0.22	73.4	47.2	25.2	268		42.4	13.0	44.6
1980	9.4	2,230	106	46.8	39.6	11.3	0.24	72.7	46.7	26.0	264		42.6	13.0	44.4
1981	9.3	2,210	104	45.6	38.9	11.4	0.25	71.5	45.6	25.9	264		42.2	12.9	44.9
1982	9.1	2,180	103	44.4	38.7	12.1	0.27	70.0	44.8	25.2	258		42.6	12.9	44.5
1983	9.0	2,140	101	44.5	37.0	12.8	0.29	69.7	44.1	25.6	253		42.6	13.0	44.3
1984	8.7	2,060	97	41.9	35.1	12.7	0.30	67.6	42.4	25.2	246		42.3	13.1	44.6
1985	8.5	2,020	96	40.6	34.7	13.1	0.32	67.4	41.9	25.5	238		42.6	13.3	44.1
1986	8.7	2,070	98	40.6	35.8	14.3	0.35	69.3	42.9	26.4	244	13.0	42.6	13.4	44.0
1987	8.6	2,040	96	39.4	34.8	14.5	0.36	68.7	42.4	26.3	241	12.7	42.2	13.5	44.3
1988	8.4	2,000	93	38.3	33.8	14.2	0.37	67.8	41.9	25.9	237	12.5	42.0	13.6	44.4
1989	8.1	1,940	90	36.9	33.1	13.6	0.37	65.9	40.8	25.0	230	12.4	41.9	13.6	44.5
1990	7.9	1,872	86	34.6	31.8	13.9	0.40	63.1	38.7	24.4	224	12.1	41.6	13.5	44.9
1991	7.8	1,840	85	33.7	31.5	13.8	0.41	62.3	38.3	24.0	223	12.2	41.4	13.3	45.3
1992	7.8	1,860	86	33.6	31.8	14.4	0.43	62.8	38.6	24.2	222	12.0	41.7	13.5	44.8

Source: MAFF: National Food Survey

Table C.2 *Consumption of milk (g/day) by type*

Year	Whole milk*	Skimmed and semi-skimmed milk	Total liquid milk
1942	291	–	291
1943	329	–	329
1944	332	–	332
1945	343	–	343
1946	330	–	330
1947	322	–	322
1948	336	–	336
1949	364	–	364
1950	399	–	364
1951	410	–	410
1952	403	–	403
1953	399	–	399
1954	402	–	402
1955	402	–	402
1956	404	–	404
1957	404	–	404
1958	401	–	401
1959	398	–	398
1960	404	–	404
1961	410	–	410
1962	414	–	414
1963	416	–	416
1964	405	–	405
1965	405	–	405
1966	412	–	412
1967	409	–	409
1968	403	–	403
1969	409	–	409
1970	387	–	387
1971	396	–	396
1972	386	1	387
1973	397	1	398
1974	396	1	3971
1975	398	1	399
1976	394	1	394
1977	379	2	381
1978	371	2	373
1979	360	3	363
1980	348	3	351
1981	335	6	341
1982	330	7	337
1983	318	10	328
1984	302	28	329
1985	277	36	313
1986	254	59	313
1987	241	65	306
1988	221	78	299
1989	202	91	293
1990	181	104	286
1991	162	114	277
1992	146	142	288

Source: MAFF: National Food Survey
• Includes school and welfare milk. Figures may not add up due to rounding.

Figure C.1: The percentage of food energy from fat in various countries (1988)

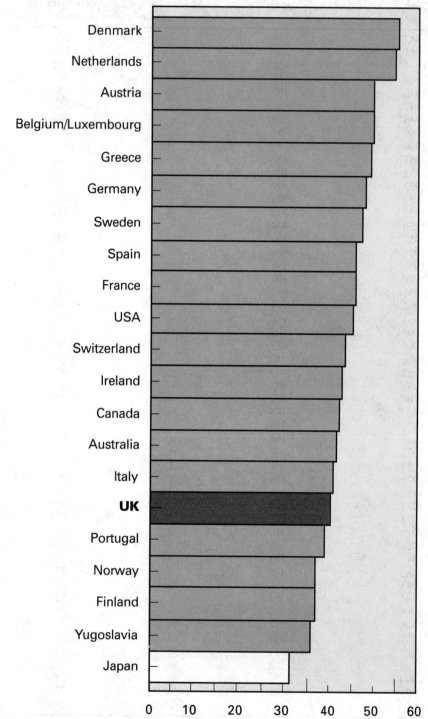

Source: Calculated by MAFF from OECD Food Consumption Statistics[32]

Printed in the United Kingdom for HMSO
Dd 299993   11/94   C40   65536   305679   44/31413